CONTENTS

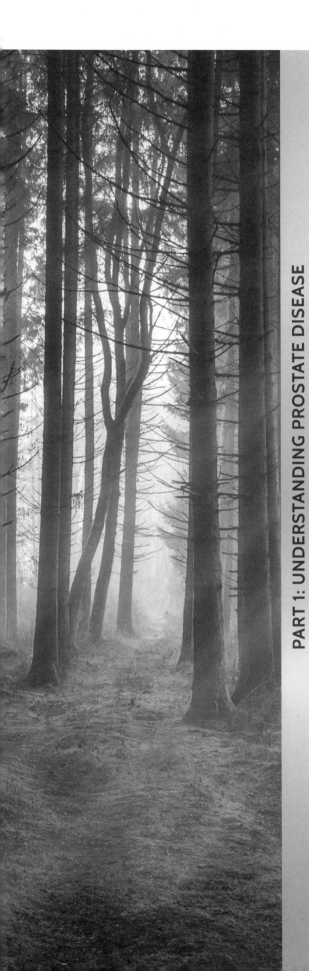

PART 1: UNDERSTANDING PROSTATE DISEASE

D1178071

CONTENTS

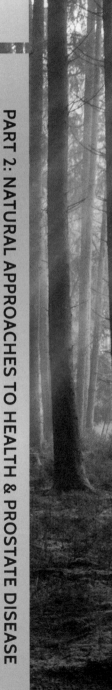

PART 2: NATURAL APPROACHES TO HEALTH & PROSTATE DISEASE

CONTENTS

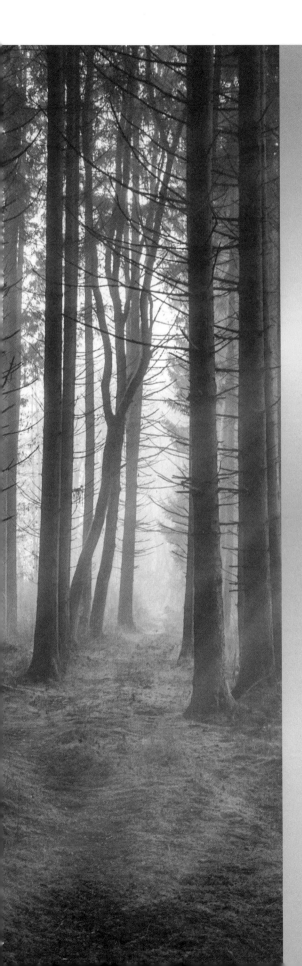

CONTENTS

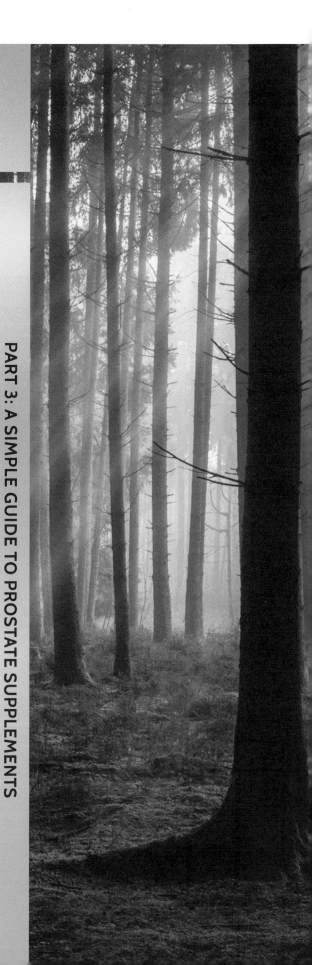

PART 3: A SIMPLE GUIDE TO PROSTATE SUPPLEMENTS

CONTENTS

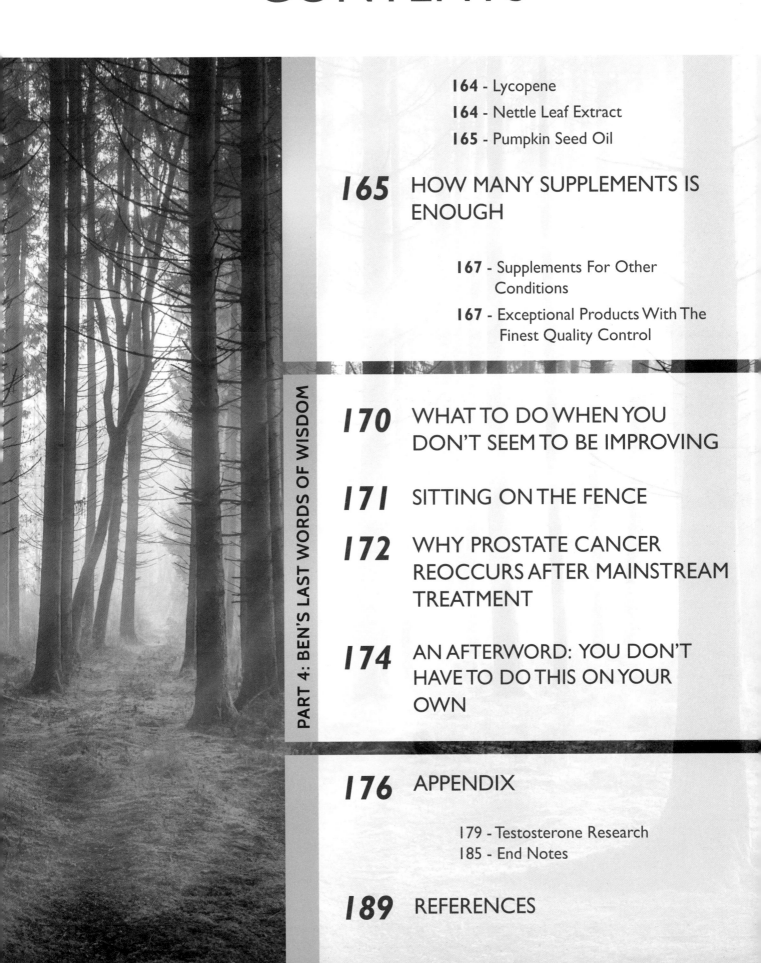

PART 1:

Understanding Prostate Disease

INTRODUCTION

Twenty years ago, I was on the cusp of retirement when my doctor told me I had prostate disease. He then told me I had to have surgery and take drugs to deal with it. I knew there had to be a better way. With a staunch belief in "food as medicine," I started right then and there researching nutrition and the prostate. I changed my diet and lifestyle pretty dramatically, and I had good results. It was then that I became curious about how these changes might affect other men. I conducted even more extensive research, interviewed numerous naturopaths, and visited clinics across the world to expand my knowledge about prostate health and the role nutrition and lifestyle play. And for the past two decades, I have worked with tens of thousands of men, helping them to improve their prostate health—and with that, their overall health! You're looking at the culmination of those two decades of work in this 10TH edition of All about the Prostate. My objective here is to give you the information you need to keep your prostate healthy, and if you are already struggling with prostate disease, to become informed about how to heal it, naturally, effectively, and quickly.

Over these years of keeping a steady pulse on the clinical research and advising other men who have one form or another of prostate disease, I think I have a pretty good grasp on what works and what doesn't. My experience has led me to conclude that virtually all the conventional medical treatments for prostate disease are in the category of things that do not work. I want to set that viewpoint straight right here. It is my opinion that pharmaceuticals (drugs) and invasive (surgical) treatments for diseases of the prostate do not work.

And there's plenty of research to back up this conclusion, which I will outline in this guide. One example of this supportive research comes from the Institute for Clinical and Economic Review (ICER) at Massachusetts General Hospital's Institute for Technology Assessment. Researchers determined in 2013 that for low-risk, localized prostate cancer in men 65 and older, observation (active surveillance [AS] or watchful waiting [WW]) was more effective than surgery and radiation therapy.

According to this ICER study, observation resulted in better quality-adjusted life-years and a comparable "net health benefit," which is short for saying nothing lost by not treating. Other studies concur. The benefits of active surveillance were confirmed in the Journal of Clinical Oncology in January 2010 and in a follow-up report in European Urology in 2011, as well as in the Journal of Clinical Oncology in December 2014. Active surveillance is akin to doing nothing at all, except your physician may want to do follow-up testing to keep an eye on your prostate condition. At any rate, what this medical research is saying is that in older men with low-risk prostate cancer, doing nothing produces better results than carrying out conventional medical treatments.

You may well wonder if what I am telling you is true, and if so, then why is it that doctors persist with all these treatments? A simple answer is that medical orthodoxy is very slow to change. What happens in clinical practice is often slow to pick up on and follow the latest research.

It could also be that prostate cancer is big business. Doctors, surgeons, hospitals, and pharmaceutical corporations are all part of a complex flow of dollars, and none of them has incentive to stop that flow. I don't mean to suggest ill-will on the part of healthcare providers. It is simply true that money matters in how diseases are treated. New studies suggest a relationship between the kinds of drugs doctors proscribe and the benefits they receive from drug companies (in the form of meals, speaking engagements, and so on). Doctors may not intentionally favor the drugs from companies offering these benefits, but the evidence is there to suggest that MDs are very likely to keep proscribing those particular drugs as long as drug companies keep marketing them with incentives to doctors. As long as the healthcare system works this way, it behooves us to not only educate ourselves about our bodies, but also to make our health priority #1.

The reality is that by the time you begin to have symptoms of prostate disease, you are already decades into problems. For many, if not most of us, these problems can be traced back to poor diet and the modern lifestyle, which doesn't mean we can't make significant changes to boost our health. Quite the contrary.

I don't want to oversimplify the matter, but as this guide will show, good nutrition and healthy lifestyle choices are crucial for prostate health. Prostate disease is a condition that happens over time, which means that fairly simple precautions can, in most cases, prevent deterioration of prostate health. Yes, it is possible to prevent prostate disease and even sometimes reverse it once it has set in by simply making a few changes in your diet, adding a few natural supplements, and making some shifts in your lifestyle. In other words, the changes called for in this guide are not beyond your reach.

The truth is, the way the healthcare system is set up now, doctors are often so busy that they have little time to sit and answer patients' questions in depth. And most of them have very little to no knowledge about nutrition. Sure, they know the basics about proteins, fats, carbohydrates, vitamins, and minerals, and that the body needs these basics to survive. But the vast majority of doctors have no idea about nutrients and how they work together to support a healthy body. Even fewer doctors have any idea how good nutrition can help with prostate disease.

I've studied nutrition in depth, and as a nutritionist, I have talked to many thousands of men who are concerned about their prostate. After implementing my advice about what and how to eat, and adding supplements, these men have consistently seen an improvement in their prostate health—and their overall health. I want to emphasize this last point. The changes I recommend in this guide, while they are directed at prostate health, positively affect your overall health. When you are eating well and making lifestyle choices that support your well-being, your whole body is positively impacted.

So, let's talk for a moment about who will benefit from reading this latest edition of All about the Prostate. Men over 50 will find this guide to be invaluable, particularly those of you who are getting up in the night multiple times to go to the toilet—a first symptom that your prostate health is deteriorating. It will also be an essential resource for those of you who have already been diagnosed with prostate disease, like an enlarged prostate, which your doctor may have called BPH (benign prostatic hyperplasia). Or perhaps you, or someone close to you, has prostate cancer. If so, don't put this book down. Read on. Anyone with these problems needs health-promoting, preventive measures NOW. It's not too late. This guide is focused on prevention, but these preventive measures are also supportive for anyone struggling with prostate disease.

A word of caution: if you are convinced that your doctor always knows best or that mainstream medicine is the most effective way to deal with prostate issues, you may find that some of the contents and research that I cite in this guide challenge your view. For instance, you'll see how strongly I challenge the mainstream medical belief that high levels of testosterone cause prostate disease. If you find yourself wondering if what I say about testosterone is credible, or if this information piques your interest and you want to learn more, then make sure to check out the appendix at the end of this guide. I've included over 60 studies that support my concerns about this medical dogma on testosterone. No matter what your views are at this moment, I encourage you to read this entire guide. Even if you favor conventional medical treatment for prostate disease, you will still find crucial information about how a good diet, lifestyle, and alternative approaches can work in tandem with, and perhaps even augment, a mainstream medical approach.

My aim is to give you the information you need to make educated decisions about your prostate health. Throughout this guide, you will find detailed information on the research that informs the opinions expressed here. It is no small task to read and absorb everything in this guide. And it may seem daunting at first to imagine making all the diet and lifestyle changes that you will find on these pages, but don't worry. This approach is not an all-or-nothing method. Just by taking a few of the steps that I suggest here, you can start your journey towards better prostate health. For now, though, all you have to do is read on!

A FEW EARLY WORDS ABOUT PROSTATE DISEASE

Before we dive into exploring the prostate and the diseases that can afflict this important gland, and later, natural methods for addressing prostate health, I want to offer a few cautionary words about the nature of conventional medicine as it is today. The truth is that doctors are trained to treat disease—not health. You go to the doctor when you have a problem. The doctor's job then is to treat that problem. Let's suppose though that you do go to the doctor without a problem. You are no more likely at this visit to hear that you should change your diet to avoid prostate cancer than you are to make an appointment for the problem you don't have! Getting advice about diet or lifestyle in advance of a problem is simply not how conventional medicine works.

Bear in mind also that the National Academy of Sciences only asks that doctors get 25 hours of nutritional training over their whole schooling. The majority of US medical schools don't offer anything close to that number. Let's think about this for a minute. It is true that younger doctors are more aware now than ever of the negative consequences of poor diet. They will now admit that poor nutrition is the prime cause of many diseases, and that includes prostate disease, but their first approach remains that of picking out a drug for you.

The food we eat makes up all the tissues of our body. Therefore, if the key to your prostate health is nutrition, and I believe it is, then how can we rely on advice that doesn't have as a solid foundation the value of nutrition? This is not to say that doctors are poorly trained or that their advice is always erroneous. I'm simply making the point that something very important is missing. The old Hippocratic adage is simple and hard to refute: "Let food be your medicine and medicine be your food."

When doctors talk about prevention, they really mean early detection. Early detection is not prevention. What's the difference? Doctors' focus on two kinds of problems: those that we complain about or those that are likely to occur as we age. They don't focus on addressing those problems until a medical test detects them. If the tests don't show a problem, then, with this approach, there's nothing wrong to treat.

I'm not making an indictment about modern medicine. Rather, I want to point to a conundrum, which is this: often issues start long before medical tests can detect them, and even long before we start having symptoms. This means that matters of health need to lean toward prevention, whereas conventional medicine is focused on detection. The two are not the same.

Detection is only helpful once disease has set in. It is the possibility of disease that makes prevention key. Really, prevention is about not taking health for granted but instead making it a priority. Even if you haven't experienced symptoms or don't have a detectable prostate issue, there are many steps you can take to ensure you don't develop a problem. And if problems have set in, then there are still changes you can make to restore health, particularly when these problems are in their early stages.

Mainstream medicine will generally pull from a relatively limited toolkit, typically recommending surgery, drugs, or even radiation therapy, each with significant documented side effects. Yet for many prostate conditions, the research data necessarily justify these treatments, which can cause everything from extreme discomfort to major, even life-threatening side-effects. Over many years of reading clinical studies, I have not found real proof that the conventional treatments have any effect on the eventual outcome of prostate disease, with the exception perhaps of aggressive prostate cancer. Permit me to share more about this point.

Studies show that once you reach the age of 65, there's no statistically significant decrease in life expectancy with active surveillance versus surgery for localized, non-aggressive prostate cancer. There is no evidence whatsoever that surgery for localized, non-aggressive prostate cancer improves quality-of-life. Studies suggest that between men who have had surgery and survived four years and those who have not had surgery and survived four years, quality-of-life is actually higher in those men who did not have surgery. Even worse, 1 out of 5 men will experience the onset of side effects, like impotence and incontinence, within two years of surgery, and often immediately afterwards.

Bear in mind that I am referring to localized, non-aggressive prostate cancer. This means the tumor is confined to the prostate. There are no metastases to the surrounding lymph nodes or other areas of the body. Aggressive prostate cancer is a different story, and we will discuss its challenges in this guide as well.

Even more problematic is when doctors recommend surgery to treat BPH (an enlarged prostate), which isn't cancer. (I'll discuss specific diseases of the prostate in a later section.) Not only does surgery not solve the problem of BPH, but it can bring on a host of side effects. And, in many cases, BPH comes back after surgery. When studies report on the efficacy of treatments, they consider what are referred to as "biomarkers," such as PSA (protein specific antigen). They are looking for whether it is going up or down as a result of a treatment. But those effects are not much help to someone with the disease if—as appears to be the case—the outcome remains much the same. In other words, many of the treatments for prostate enlargement offer only temporary changes but little long-term effect on the actual disease process

I have talked extensively to men grappling with prostate disease—and by this, I mean, enlarged prostate (BPH), prostate infection or inflammation (prostatitis), and localized, as well as invasive prostate cancer. Each of them has discovered the same thing: prostate health is directly linked to quality-of-life. The symptoms of prostate disease effect so many aspects of your life. If you wake several times a night to urinate, you will not get good quality sleep, so you will feel tired, weak, and older than you are. Plus, you will not benefit from the restorative aspects of sleep that actually help us heal. The impairment to your sexual function will rob you of a fulfilling romantic life and may make you feel lesser, embarrassed, and unmanly. The risk of public incontinence will rob you of your freedom and force you to avoid going to places that are too far from easily accessible bathrooms. More than anything, men who are faced with prostate disease soon realize that this tiny gland that they had ignored all their life is vitally important to their longevity, their health, and their happiness.

That's why every man I speak to has been trying to do something about it. Some have followed mainstream medical treatment, and some have used natural approaches. Some men try to cover their bases by doing both. My experience tells me that those going the natural route seem to have a safer, more pleasant experience with fewer, if any side effects. This means less treatment-related pain, incontinence, and impotence, to name just a few side effects.

And, from the feedback I have received over the years, natural treatment seems to be at least as effective as conventional medicine when it comes to many of the diseases of the prostate, certainly when it comes to an enlarged prostate. By natural treatment, I mean a prostate-health-specific diet, lifestyle habits (exercise, stress-management practices, restorative sleep, reducing toxin overload), and the addition of nutrient-packed dietary supplements. Many men who choose the natural route for benign diseases of the prostate experience positive changes just as frequently, if not more so, than men going the conventional medical route. These include lower PSA and a reduction in the size of the prostate and the symptoms associated with prostate disease.

The benefits to a natural approach are numerous. Foremost, the objective of the natural route is to get at the cause of the disease. I want to emphasize here that the natural approach tends to go to the source and not the symptom. Going straight to the source is, in my opinion, far better than short-term symptom reduction from pharmaceuticals that bring with them plenty of side effects. Not only that, many men lose weight from the diet changes and regular exercise that I outline in this guide. A healthy weight is clearly linked to increased longevity, lower risk of heart disease, and increased mental sharpness, amongst other effects. Moreover, some dietary supplements, such as those with ingredients found in Ben's Natural Health supplements, provide additional benefits that extend well beyond those related to the prostate. I will go into more detail about supplements later.

When comparing both ways of going about treating prostate disease—conventional medicine versus an integrative, natural approach—I admit freely that my experience gives me a personal bias towards the natural route. I have experienced the benefits and I have seen them in countless numbers of men. That said, for you to have all the information you need to make educated decisions about your health, this guide will detail mainstream treatments and provide a comprehensive natural approach to fostering prostate health.

The bottom line about taking steps to prevent prostate disease is that this comprehensive program that I outline really works. It will also impact your overall health positively. More than that: prostate disease can often be reversed—even localized, non-aggressive prostate cancer.

If you neglect your symptoms though, not only will a problem get worse over time, but other complications can set in. For instance, if it's difficult to pass water, for men over 50 at least, this usually means the prostate is enlarged. If you ignore the fact that you are waking multiple times at night to go to the toilet, then you are also ignoring the possibility that backward pressure may be starting to develop, first on your bladder, and then on your kidney. You might think of this scenario as one of having too much water behind the dam, and it just keeps backing up. Not only is there a problem with your prostate gland in this situation, but a whole cascade of problems starts to occur: first, the bladder gets irritated and then infected and soon after, so do your kidneys. Kidneys are very sensitive organs that can be easily damaged, and irreversibly so, by this kind of back-up pressure.

Pay attention to symptoms when they arise. Ignoring symptoms is never a good idea.

You will find detailed information in this guide about eliminating the source of prostate problems, with a lot of emphasis on diet changes geared toward reducing inflammation, boosting the immune system, and balancing the sex hormones—all of which benefit the prostate! You will also find extensive information about diet and natural supplements to support a healthy prostate, as well as detailed suggestions about making a healthy lifestyle, through regular exercise and managing the inevitability of stress. But first, I want to walk you through the information you need to know about the prostate and its healthy functioning, and what happens when it starts to show signs of disease, as well as how conventional medicine treats these diseases.

A HEALTHY PROSTATE & ITS FUNCTIONS

Typically, men begin to pay attention to their prostate only when something goes wrong. Alternatively, after a certain age, a prostate exam becomes part of a regular physical exam. But to know how to care for the prostate before then, it's a good idea to know a little bit about what it is and does.

A healthy prostate weighs about three-fourths of an ounce (20 grams) and is approximately the size of a walnut. It surrounds and envelops the urethra (the tube that carries urine from the bladder through the penis) and sits just beneath the bladder. A healthy prostate has a smooth, soft surface and a firm but springy feel to it. A doctor will often feel for hardness, lumps, nodules, and lesions to determine if the prostate is diseased or potentially cancerous. So, what does the prostate do?

1. Its main function is to secrete prostatic fluids, which help nourish, liquify, and protect sperm. The prostate gland and these fluids are therefore vitally important for ensuring fertility. The fluid excreted by the prostate contributes about a third of the total volume of the ejaculated semen and is made up of various enzymes, minerals, and other nutrients.

One notable component of prostatic fluid is the protein, prostate specific antigen (PSA). I'm sure you have heard of PSA. This protein's job is to liquefy semen; it works to prevent thickening after ejaculation. The thinning action allows sperm to swim more freely and aids in fertility. *Protein*

A small amount of the PSA naturally makes its way into your blood stream. A PSA test measures the amount of PSA in the blood. The larger the prostate the more PSA it produces and therefore, the more PSA that will make its way into your blood. Prostate cancer cells also produce PSA. In fact, cancer cells produce more PSA than a healthy prostate does, and this is why a high PSA level is correlated with the likelihood of prostate cancer. Obviously, the PSA test is not perfect. You can have a low PSA but still have prostate cancer or a high PSA and no prostate cancer. For these reasons, it's best to think of the PSA test as a general indicator, at best, of prostate health.

Enzyme

2. The prostate gland is also one of the places that the body produces a crucial enzyme called 5-alpha-reductase. This enzyme converts the male sexual hormone, testosterone, to dihydrotestosterone (DHT), which is anywhere from five to ten times more powerful than regular testosterone. DHT seems to have a wide range of impacts across the body, particularly the initial growth of the prostate during adolescence, although scientists are still unsure of all its purposes. What we do know is that DHT is one of the primary hormones contributing to masculine features and traits that appear during puberty. We also know that it plays a vital role in managing male sex drive. Studies have linked DHT to cognitive ability, heart health, memory, and even blood sugar levels.

Enzyme = Hormone

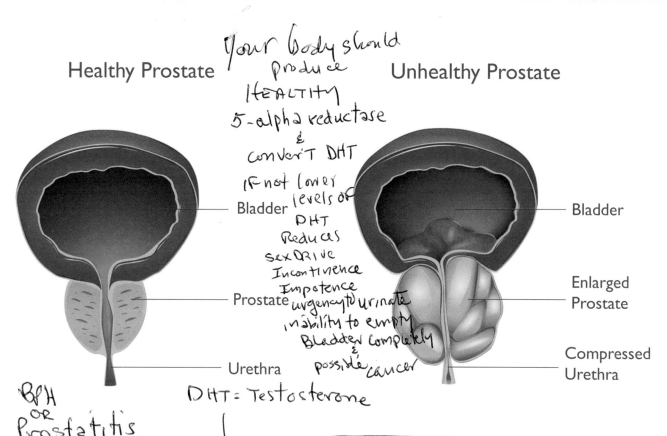

Healthy Prostate   Unhealthy Prostate

Bladder

Prostate

Urethra

Bladder

Enlarged Prostate

Compressed Urethra

Handwritten notes:

Your body should produce HEALTHY 5-alpha reductase & convert DHT

If not lower levels of DHT Reduces sex DRIVE Incontinence Impotence urgency to urinate inability to empty Bladder completely & possible cancer

BPH OR Prostatitis

DHT = Testosterone

What does this mean for you? Well, if your prostate becomes enlarged (also known as benign prostatic hyperplasia [BPH]) or inflamed or infected (called prostatitis), for example, then your body's ability to produce 5-alpha-reductase and convert testosterone to DHT may become impaired. We know that lower DHT levels may reduce your sex drive. But a declining sex drive is just one of a host of problems that can occur. Incontinence, impotence, urgency to urinate, an inability to empty your bladder completely, and in the longer run, a higher risk of cancer can all stem from an enlarged prostate, which, my experience tells me, is an easily reversible problem.

DISEASES OF THE PROSTATE

The odds are 2:1 that, for those of you reading this guide—which means that you are likely based either in the United States or Europe—by the time you turn 60, you will have experienced some form of a prostate problem. Another way of looking at it is that if you eat a typical Western diet and live a typically modern life, you only have a 1-in-3 chance of avoiding a prostate issue before you turn 60. Those odds shrink as you age. These problems include prostatitis (when the prostate gland becomes inflamed or infected), enlargement of the prostate (BPH), localized, non-invasive prostate cancer, and finally, though far less frequently, invasive, metastatic cancer of the prostate.

Let's go straight to the issue of cancer and work our way back, because if we're honest, it's cancer that terrifies most of us, and for good reason. But what I hope you will understand by the time you finish this guide, and even this section, is that the best way to think of prostate disease is as a continuum with cancer at the far end. Now, it is not apparent that this is the case always, but bear with me for a bit while I explain. First though, the cancer question: professor Jane Plant gives us a good start in her book, Prostate Cancer: Understand, Prevent and Overcome. She writes:

"Interpretation of the data is complicated ... by the extent to which some prostate cancers are slow growing and cause no problems during a normal lifetime while others are potentially life-threatening-metastasis cancers. From autopsies performed on men who have died of other causes, it is known that small amounts of cancer can be found within the prostates of many men. These lesions can first be detected shortly after the onset of puberty, with the frequency increasing steadily with age. By the time men reach the age of 70 and above, 80–100 percent will have such lesions. While these numbers are high, only approximately 0.3% of these patients will develop metastatic prostate cancer in any given year. Because it is only metastatic prostate cancer that is potentially lethal, it is important to understand what stimulates cancer to spread beyond the confines of the gland."

Dr. Plant's insistence on the need to understand the conditions that cause prostate cancer to worsen and spread, or even the conditions that contribute to having prostate cancer in the first place is what I hope the pages that follow will show. But let's talk numbers and percentages briefly, to put some things in perspective.

Globally, prostate cancer is the third most common cancer, after lung and breast, and the most common cancer among men over 65. Of all the cancer diagnoses in men over the age of 65 in Europe and the US, 80% of the time it's prostate cancer. Approximately 165,000 men in the US are diagnosed with prostate cancer each year, which means that about 3.1 million men in the US are living with this disease. The majority of those cancers are localized. Localized, non-aggressive cancers are not invasive or metastasizing (spreading to other parts of the body). And of those men diagnosed with localized prostate cancer, over 98% survive at least 10 years.

Now, let's talk about the real scare: death. In the United States, prostate cancer is the second leading cause of cancer death. But this statistic can be misleading. Fewer than 30,000 men in the US die each year from prostate cancer. This number amounts to about 1% of the 3.1 million men living with the disease—and almost 90% of those men are over the age of 65. Recall that the older you are, the more likely you are to develop prostate disease, which also means prostate cancer. In general, 1 in 21 men between the ages of 60 and 65 develop invasive prostate cancer, whereas 1 in 12 men 70 and older develop this disease. Only 80 out of 1 million men in the US will have metastases to the lymph nodes, which is when the cancer is more likely to spread and become deadly.

What do all of these numbers tell us? Well, let me first say that I'm not jumping to discuss death to create a scare—quite the opposite, in fact. I want you to know that prostate cancer is incredibly common, and more often than not, the cancer is non-invasive and slow-growing. We'll talk more about how prostate cancer is classified into localized, non-invasive or invasive subtypes in the section on tests, but for those of you who are 70 and older, the statistics illustrate that prostate cancer is not likely to be the cause of your death.

I want to shift back now to other prostate diseases, keeping in mind this idea of a continuum. But let's be cautious in not jumping immediately to the idea that one problem causes another. Researchers are very careful about linking prostate problems in this way, but I'm of the perspective that prostate disease is like a spectrum of worsening problems that are all related.

We'll begin with prostatitis, which, as I have offered, is the medical term for an infected or inflamed prostate. When younger men (under the age of 45) experience prostatitis, they typically experience it as an isolated event that doesn't recur. For older men, however, prostatitis can be recurrent and chronic. The cause of prostatitis is usually some type of bacterial or viral infection, but not always. Sometimes it is not clear what is causing the inflammation and/or infection. Men with prostatitis complain of back pain, pain with emptying the bladder, discomfort with ejaculation, and aching in the pelvic floor.

BPH (benign prostatic hyperplasia) is the most common condition of the prostate. It rarely occurs in men under the age of 40. Approximately half of men over 65 in the UK and a similar percentage (around 15 million men) in the United States are diagnosed annually with BPH. This number doesn't include all of the men who have symptoms but who have as yet decided against going to the doctor, either ignoring the problem or treating it in their own way.

BPH occurs when the prostate gland becomes enlarged, and hard nodules form on the gland. When this enlargement or these nodules encroach upon the urethra and bladder due to the limited amount of space in the region of the prostate, men experience all kinds of symptoms related to passing urine: an urgent need to go, waking in the night to pee, sometimes several times, difficulty starting the flow of urine, a feeling of not finishing urinating, weak flow, and dribbling. Because the flow of urine slows and/or gets backed up, BPH also tends to cause other problems like UTIs (urinary tract infections). These problems can eventually lead to kidney infections and other problems of the kidneys.

BPH = Enlarged prostate

An enlarged prostate can also lead to prostatitis, and for the past several decades researchers have been looking into a link between BPH and prostate cancer. While these researchers are hesitant to say definitively that BPH causes prostate cancer, they have been willing to suggest that there is a link. Some wonder if both are caused by inflammation. The plot thickens, then, because we have already said that healthy diet and lifestyle can go a long way in preventing the deterioration of prostate health—and many of the suggestions in this guide are aimed at reducing inflammation in the body, which also means, of the prostate.

To recap, there are basically three prostate diagnoses that encompass prostate disease: prostatitis (infection/inflammation), BPH (enlarged prostate), and prostate cancer (diagnosed along a graded spectrum from local, slow-growing and non-invasive to more aggressive, invasive, and metastasizing). The symptoms for these problems, as we shall see, are similar. Importantly, if you are having symptoms now, you've got a problem that has been in the making for some time. But this is not reason to fear. The important thing to know is that there is a lot you can do to help your prostate.

SYMPTOMS OF PROSTATE DISEASE

Many men are in denial that they may have a problem because they believe that getting up at night is an inevitable part of growing older. It's not. Getting up multiple times in the night to go to the bathroom is the earliest symptom of a brewing prostate problem.

Other men experience discomfort, burning, or chronic pain in the pelvic floor, difficulty starting to urinate, a weak stream, urgency and a feeling of not being able to completely empty the bladder, and dribbling after or in between urinating. This combination of urinary symptoms is often referred to as lower urinary tract symptoms or LUTS. Some studies report that more than 50% of men age 50 and older also experience erectile dysfunction or ED. This percentage goes up with increasing age. Studies also make a direct link between the development of ED with prostate enlargement and LUTS. ED negatively effects quality-of-life and can lead to depression. But depression, stress, and relationship problems can also contribute to ED separate from prostate problems, as can health-depleting lifestyle choices like cigarette smoking. Conventional medical treatments, as I indicate below, can also cause or worsen ED.

All that notwithstanding, many men with prostate disease experience ED, loss of libido, and lack of male energy. These symptoms are not an inevitable part of aging. Nor are they something to just live with, despite the fact that having sexual problems can be degrading and embarrassing to confront. Studies show that the overwhelming majority of men with sexual problems do not mention them or seek help, but I am here to tell you that they are symptoms of prostate disease and can be remedied with the right support and plan of action.

Still other men get notifications from their doctors that their PSA levels have gone up significantly. Western doctors often encourage the belief that a rise in PSA levels signals a problem with the prostate. Elevated PSA levels do not necessarily mean that a man has prostate disease. It could signal a problem, but maybe not. Just because prostate disease happens to be almost universal in the western world does not make it inevitable. This point cannot be overemphasized: prostate disease is not inevitable.

That said, I do not want to downplay the seriousness of prostate disease. As I iterate a number of times in this guide: if BPH is left untreated, the result can be repeated UTIs (urinary tract infections) and bladder infections, and even kidney infections, the eventual need for a catheter, and impotence. Not only that, untreated BPH can cause a great deal of pain.

It is an old truism that an ounce of prevention is better than a pound of cure. If you are already experiencing the early symptoms of prostate disease, then getting your prostate back to good health is not only critical for you now, but it's also not that difficult. From my experience, diet is key. Knowing which foods to eat and which ones to avoid is paramount to helping reverse prostate disease and to preventing disease in the first place. The same is true about adding exercise, managing stress and exposure to environmental toxins, and boosting good nutrition with natural food supplements.

WHAT CAUSES PROSTATE DISEASE?

As with all chronic diseases, there are a number of factors that combine to cause prostate disease. We often hear about genetic predisposition. Clearly, you cannot change the genes you inherit—at least not yet—but our DNA, in any event, only contributes to susceptibility. It's not written in stone that we will or will not develop the problem we are predisposed to. In other words, our genes are not "fixed." They change based on how we live our lives: by what we eat, drink, how much we move and sleep, and how we respond to stress. Similarly, environmental factors can contribute over the long haul to the development of prostate disease. There are changes that we can make to alter at least some of the environmental factors that can contribute to disease. These include air and food quality. Even sound and light pollution can trigger the stress response or negatively affect the quality of our sleep. What may seem like insignificant stressors can set into motion a long cascade of responses in our body that, over time, can negatively affect our health. Many of these stressors rev up the inflammatory processes and challenge immune systems. And on it goes until, eventually, we've got a problem—unless we intervene and make our health priority #1.

This little excerpt on lifestyle is not intended to oversimplify by saying that preventing and treating prostate disease is simply a matter of living right. Rather, I'm saying that we need to look at prostate disease—like so many chronic diseases—as a sign of bodily wear and tear. With that said, and bearing in mind that in so many respects, our lives are in our own hands, let us look more closely at some of the factors that cause problems with the prostate gland.

INFLAMMATION

Simply put, anything that irritates the prostate leads to inflammation of the prostate, which, over the long term, contributes to prostate disease. That's a plain way of saying that chronic, systemin inflammation and prostate disease go hand-in-hand.

It should come as no surprise to you by now for me to say that certain foods can cause major irritation to your prostate because they contribute to chronic inflammation throughout the body, including the prostate gland. Suffice it to say early on that processed foods, refined sugar, dairy, and caffeine all have a direct impact on your prostate. I have devoted a whole section to diet in Part 2, but I want to emphasize here that one of the leading causes of chronic inflammation stems from what we eat.

Inflammation takes place when the body is trying to repair damage. When we have an injury or infection, the immune system responds to this injury via inflammatory chain reactions that serve to heal the injured or damaged tissues. This scenario is that of acute inflammation.

Inflammation becomes a problem when it goes on for too long and becomes chronic. In the prostate gland, the inflammatory processes cause cells to multiply and change the way genes get expressed. Multiplying cells can contribute to enlargement of the prostate, and changes in genes can contribute to cancer. The point is that chronic inflammation in the prostate can signal reactions that, over time, contribute to prostate disease in one form or another.

Direct pressure is also irritating to the prostate gland, likely caused by reduced blood flow in the area. When blood flow is reduced for too long, the immune system sends out an inflammatory response to repair the tissues that are not getting enough oxygen. Too frequent or chronic pressure on the pelvic floor can cause this inflammation to become chronic. Cycling or sitting on a seat that doesn't properly support the whole pelvis can cause these kinds of reactions. In fact, cyclists who trained for more than four hours a week were found to be six times more likely to have prostate issues than those who didn't.

HORMONES (BUT NOT TESTOSTERONE!)

Hormones can also be irritating to the prostate, specifically DHT (dihydrotestosterone) and estrogens. We discussed DHT briefly in the section on the prostate and its functions. As I pointed out there, DHT is the highly active form of testosterone that circulates in the bloodstream. Mainstream medicine wrongly believes the cause of prostate cancer is too much testosterone (not DHT), and one common hormone treatment for prostate cancer wipes out testosterone in the patient. But there is a large body of recent research that is still discounted by medical orthodoxy, which says that there is no link between testosterone and prostate cancer. This new research points instead to DHT. Understanding this hormone and its role in prostate health is important.

DHT is critical early in life. It helps to differentiate and develop male genitalia in the embryo. It is also critical in puberty for its role in the growth and maturation of the penis, scrotum, and the body as a whole—the muscle mass and body frame that characterize the male. It also contributes to the development of facial, body, and pubic hair, and a deeper voice.

As we age, DHT can overpower decreasing levels of testosterone. At the same time, estrogen (female hormones) production starts to increase relative to testosterone. Don't worry, every man and woman have testosterone and estrogen. It is the proper balance of the two hormones that keeps men and women healthy. But, in the West, by the age of 55 most men have more estrogens in their bloodstream than their wives do! This change in hormonal balance seems to be a key element in the development of prostate disease, although the role this imbalance plays in prostate disease is still not clear.

Some researchers suggest that too much estrogen can trigger inflammation in the prostate. What we do know is that when the ratio of estrogen to testosterone rises, the body responds by converting some testosterone to DHT. When this happens, prostate cells are likely to start growing, because we know that DHT stimulates the growth of the prostate. So, the combination of too much estrogen with elevated DHT seems to irritate the prostate. What can be done?

Certain factors can increase estrogen production in men. The most significant contributing factor is animal fats, and none more so than dairy. The average diet in the West contains a massively higher proportion of dairy than diets in the East. Studies have looked at the relationship between dairy consumption and cancer rates, so much so that researchers have started to pay attention to the differences not only in consumption of milk between different cultures and how these differences relate to the incidence of cancers. They have also started to look at the differences between the milk produced from commercial dairy cows and that of more traditionally raised cows. It turns out that commercial dairy is much higher in estrogen than milk from cows raised and milked the old-fashioned way. What is significant about these studies is that they make a direct correlation between dairy intake and cancer, prostate cancer being one of them.

For aging men whose hormones are already prone to imbalance, this means consuming dairy is a strong risk factor for prostate disease. But we have established that prostate disease is a chronic disease that starts long before symptoms are noticeable. So, younger men are not off the hook when it comes to drinking milk!

Also, sedentary men who do not get vigorous exercise produce less testosterone. This combination of a diet high in animal fat plus little or no exercise describes the diet and lifestyle of most western men. This combination ultimately leads to an increase in the ratio of estrogen to testosterone as men age, and we have seen already what this imbalance can do.

Why Mainstream Medicine Continues to Insist That Testosterone is the Cause of Prostate Disease

A lot of men have come to me saying they've been offered a treatment that doesn't involve surgery. Their urologist has told them that by getting rid of their testosterone, they can remove the risk of prostate cancer, with none of the side effects of surgery. There's a problem with this line of reasoning. Hormone therapy can cause quite a few side effects, so just because it's not surgery doesn't mean that hormone therapy is side-effect free.

The most pressing concern is the idea that testosterone is "bad" for your prostate and that it makes prostate cancer grow. This idea, as I started to show above, is just plain erroneous and is part of a mainstream medical dogma that persists, despite quite a lot of research to the contrary. For the past almost eighty years, the idea that testosterone causes prostate cancer has pervaded conventional medicine's approach to treating prostate disease. But, get this: the fall in testosterone as men age almost exactly parallels the rise in incidence of BPH, prostatitis, and prostate cancer. If testosterone alone was the cause of prostate cancer, then 18-year-old men—who have the highest levels of testosterone—would suffer from prostate cancer. Of course they don't. Something just doesn't line up with this "high testosterone" dogma.

Curiously enough, about seventy years ago doctors had a completely different take on testosterone.

They also understood the detrimental effects of too much estrogen. And they were aware of the all-important testosterone-to-estrogen ratio. Over eighty studies were quoted on the entire subject. The medical thinking changed in the 1940s when Dr. Charles Brenton Huggins got the Nobel prize in medicine after treating prostate cancer patients by castrating them.

The table below shows the average testosterone level for your age range. Bear in mind that men fluctuate by more than 50% in either direction at each age. Still, this table can be a helpful general road map.

AGE RANGE	AVERAGE TOTAL (ng/dL)
45-49	546
50-54	544
55-64	562
65-74	524
75-84	471
85-100	376

In the Appendix at the end of this guide, I show you substantial clinical data from universities, hospitals, and clinics all over the world that confirm testosterone is not the cause of prostate disease. I am terribly concerned about the extent to which conventional medical practice can be in such direct conflict with very clear and overwhelming scientific evidence. The evidence that high levels of testosterone do not cause prostate cancer provides plenty of reason to question the practice of prescribing hormone therapy to lower testosterone levels. This type of therapy based on a false premise may seriously negatively affect the condition of your prostate.

Why this treatment protocol continues is probably multifaceted. Trends and beliefs in science and medicine are notoriously slow to change. Moving from new research to general acceptance can easily take a generation or more. A good example of this took place in the mid-1980s when new ideas surfaced about the cause of stomach ulcers. Interestingly, the man who discovered that ulcers are not the result of eating too much spicy food but are instead the result of a bacterial infection wasn't actually acknowledged until 2005 when he was awarded a Nobel prize. During those nearly 30 years, your doctor likely would have told you to eat less spicy food if you had a stomach ulcer, even though the evidence overwhelmingly pointing to bacteria as the cause had long since been published!

Reputations of senior doctors and professors often hang on their earlier conclusions, even if those conclusions are later proven to be erroneous. Such doctors and professors are not in a hurry to admit that the treatments, which made their reputation, were off-base. It is important to recognize here that doctors and researchers can and sometimes do lose their jobs if they insist on breaching the prevailing common consensus. The medical establishment itself, along with insurance companies and pharmaceutical corporations (who singularly and altogether have a lot of power) have a vested interest in maintaining the status quo. Medical history is full of instances of researchers who have been sent into the medical wilderness only to have their views confirmed many years later.

I often say that when trying to understand any field, a good rule of thumb is to "follow the money." In the medical industry, it flows from two places: the pharmaceutical and the insurance corporations. Earlier, I mentioned drug corporation incentives to doctors. This influence has a serious impact on how medicine is practiced. Not only do doctors follow the models for treatment that have been made available to them, but since there is no one out there offering incentives in the direction of healing through nutrition, exercise, and lifestyle changes, doctors fall in line with the established routine dictated by a powerful pharmaceutical industry and the specific interventions that insurance companies pay for. Ironic as it may seem, insurance companies won't pay for healing through nutrition, exercise, and lifestyle changes.

Pharmaceutical corporations are certainly in no hurry to kill off very profitable drugs either—in this case, those that combat testosterone. Certainly, corporate interests and profits provide sufficient motivation to disregard inconvenient new research. Many researchers and clinicians are funded by these interests, which then bias research, either advertently or inadvertently.

Ultimately, doctors are only human. That's why it can come as a personal affront to them when new science research conflicts with what they believe. It's the reason that when Ignaz Semmelweis discovered that anyone delivering a baby should wash their hands beforehand, he was fired from the hospital where he worked and actually committed to an asylum for questioning doctor's hygiene. Not only that, even with the information and evidence that he had provided, the doctors in that Austrian hospital went back to delivering babies with the very same (unwashed!) hands they used on autopsies. And so it goes. If you want to know more about the research on testosterone and the prostate, make sure to read the Testosterone Research Appendix at the end of this guide.

PIGGY IN THE MIDDLE

It is hardly surprising that men get very confused by the conflicting messages coming from conventional medicine and natural practitioners. After all, no one seems to be able to agree about the cause of the prostate problem and how to treat it. Doctors and medical specialists have years of study with a very particular viewpoint about disease, high-tech equipment to "fix broken parts," and the support of an old establishment that comprises the history of medicine itself, along with the pervasive incentives from pharmaceutical corporations and demands for compliance from the insurance industry.

A doctor walks into the room of an ailing patient with his long white coat on, and the ailing patient is already conditioned to revere the authority of this person. The coat suggests immediately that this person a) is at the top of the hierarchy of healthcare staff in his office or hospital, and therefore, b) has had years of study, and so, c) has at his disposal, all kinds of knowledge and methods to fix any problem that has to do with the body. It is not surprising therefore that many men feel reassured by and have a lot of faith in their doctor telling them what to do.

Men who are oriented toward a natural approach as a first line of healthcare, on the other hand, may question the status quo. These men also tend to be oriented toward self-education about their bodies and take an active role in prevention. When confronted with disease, they may struggle with the choices offered by conventional medicine. Some of these men will stay away from these conventional approaches, wary of them. Others may find themselves caught between their preference for the natural approach but torn about the choices they face, fearful of the outcome of the disease and the medical treatment options. These men, I call "piggy in the middle," struggling with what they believe, all the information coming their way, and fear about their disease

To those of you seeking as much information as you can find on the internet about prostate disease, I want to issue a word of caution. While there is no doubt that the internet is a wonderful repository of information, and access to information is easier now than ever, there are some cranks out there with some pretty strange ideas, and many medical websites are not even written by a person with a medical degree or healthcare background!

Also, some websites are directly or indirectly supported by pharmaceutical corporations. These drug corporations clearly have an agenda, as does anyone who has products to sell. It could surely be said that I have an agenda by providing this guide and telling you about lifestyle changes and the products we have developed over the years. While this is so, I hope that, more than anything, you walk away from reading this guide with the information you need to make informed decisions about your health that feel right for you. I hope I have and continue to make my own personal biases clear.

Not all information is biased to the point of being wrong. I simply encourage you to be properly skeptical and make careful judgments that make sense to you and the health of your body. We have already established that pharmaceutical corporations have an overwhelming influence on the medical profession. They also have too much influence on our trust in natural approaches to health. I like to encourage all the men I speak with to bear in mind that the drug corporations make their money selling drugs that target symptoms only. Let's be honest, they profit not only when you get sick but as importantly when you stay sick. If you experience side effects, rest assured they will provide more drugs that aim to combat those too. It's a never-ending cycle, and once you're in it, you've got to work extra hard to get out. My advice is this: don't get in the pharmaceutical cycle. Take nutrition seriously, and by that, I mean the food and natural supplements that you put into your body. This one small step will completely change your life.

A final word on this topic, if you are that piggy in the middle, I encourage you not to accept anything at face value. Doing so could cost you dearly. Do continue to educate yourself. Read up on all the research and make up your own mind about what is right for you. Reading this guide is a great first step!

TEST & DIAGNOSIS

There is no one test for diagnosing prostate disease that is both substantially reliable and non-invasive. This is particularly true in the UK where the current best and safest tests are not available.

Conventional medicine relies largely on 5 tests for diagnosing prostate disease. They are:

1. Digital Rectal examination (DRE)
2. Prostate-specific antigen test (PSA)
3. Magnetic Resonance Imaging (MRI)
4. Needle biopsy
5. 3D color ultrasound, (sonogram) (not available in the UK)

A sixth, very new test, is a urine test called PCA3. The PCA3 is claimed to be more reliable than the PSA test. (For UK readers, note that the PCA3 is also not available in the UK unless you see a urologist privately.)

A number of new tests are available now, but they tend to be expensive, unfortunately, and highly specific. As a result, only a select handful of individuals can benefit from them. The only exception is the 4Kscore (also not available in the UK), which I recommend to everyone at my clinic in Arizona. Especially when used in conjunction with the other tests that form part of my Advanced Prostate Cancer Risk Assessment (APCRA), the 4Kscore is the most predictive test for prostate cancer and its potential to be life-threatening.

Finally, the APCRA that I just mentioned uses a whole range of tests and includes a Color Doppler scan. I describe this in more detail below.

Although enlargement of your prostate can start in your thirties, conventional medicine will not consider you to be at risk for prostate disease (and therefore push you toward screening) until you're in your fifties or sixties, typically. This push for screening might happen a little earlier if you are of African or Caribbean descent because of a higher incidence of prostate disease for reasons we don't understand yet. Regardless, after a certain age, a lot of doctors will add one of the following tests to your annual check-up.

The two most common tests for detecting prostate cancer and other prostate diseases are the digital rectal exam (DRE) and the prostate specific antigen test (PSA test), but I detail all of them here.

DIGITAL RECTAL EXAM (DRE)

As unpleasant as it may be or seem, a digital rectal examination (DRE) is the first and least invasive test given by a diagnostician. A DRE also has the potential to be one of the more revealing tests, but it does depend entirely on the skill of the physician doing it. A doctor will check for palpable (found by touch) abnormalities in the prostate, through the thin wall of the rectum. This palpation (examination by touch) is done with a gloved finger using a lubricant. The entire gland cannot be checked with the DRE, however, which is why other tests may also be necessary.

PROSTATE SPECIFIC ANTIGEN (PSA)

The PSA test measures the levels of prostate specific antigen in your blood. Recall that the PSA is a protein that liquefies and prevents thickening of semen after ejaculation. This thinning action allows sperm to swim more freely and aids in fertility. You will recall also that the prostate makes PSA, and prostate cancer cells make more than normal amounts of PSA, so as men age and are considered to be at higher risk for prostate cancer, MDs test for PSA levels in the blood using the PSA blood test. BPH and prostatitis can also elevate PSA levels.

As I indicated earlier, the PSA blood test is an unreliable indicator for prostate disease, in that a high score is not necessarily bad news, nor is a low score a guarantee that you don't have problems. Having one "off" test in a year might just indicate that you had an infection, drank coffee, or even that you had recently had sex—all things that can cause a short-term rise in your PSA level. What's most important to monitor is how the PSA level trends. A sudden spike, maintained over a period of 3–6 months can indicate prostatitis or cancer, while a gradual increase over a period of 18–24 months is a strong indicator of BPH. Nonetheless, the test is imprecise and needs to be verified alongside other tests.

In the last couple of years, there have been a number of more advanced versions of the PSA test that use added statistical methods. One well-known example of this is the PSA-Free test, but there are several other less well-known ones. None of these newer tests by themselves offer that much more information than the standard PSA test, with the exception of the 4Kscore, which I detail below.

BIOPSY

If your PSA level goes up over an extended period, then the next step is to get a needle biopsy of the prostate tissue. As the name suggests, a needle biopsy is the extraction of prostate tissue by means of a needle inserted into the prostate gland. Usually, your MD will order a biopsy to establish whether or not cancer is present. There are, however, various problems with a needle biopsy, and, as with the PSA test, the results may not necessarily be conclusive. A prostate biopsy will only detect prostate cancer 85% of the time. In case this is not obvious, this means that at least 15% of biopsies miss the presence of cancerous cells. There are also occasionally false-positive results that suggest cancer is there when it is not.

Also, more than 50% of men have side effects after a biopsy of the prostate. Infection is the most frequent side effect, even though antibiotics are routinely given before the procedure. What is even more concerning is the fact that if prostate cancer is present, the needle that cuts cells from the prostate becomes contaminated with cancerous cells and then, when the same needle is used in a new location of the prostate that is not cancerous, it can transfer the cancer to the new location. This process is called "needle tracking."

It takes an average of eighteen months for the newly seeded cancer to show up in any diagnostic test when needle tracking occurs. For all those reasons, I do not recommend prostate biopsy except in unusual circumstances. Nevertheless, prostate biopsy is the standard test in the US and UK for establishing the presence of cancer cells. Generally, medical insurance companies will only cover the cost of treatment for prostate cancer if there is a positive prostate biopsy result. This means also that hospitals will only provide prostate cancer treatment when a prostate biopsy produces a positive result.

The pathology report for a prostate biopsy includes what is referred to as a Gleason score. The Gleason score indicates the presence and aggressiveness of prostate cancer cells. A higher score correlates with more aggressive tumors. However, even the Gleason score can be misleading and does not conclusively establish the correct level of virulence.

Needle biopsies often lead to extremely painful, long-lasting infections, which are difficult to treat even with the strongest antibiotics. And antibiotics are problematic too! The biggest problem with them is that even when they are successful at combating an infection, they lay the groundwork for the next infection because they wipe out all the good microbes in your gut and seriously compromise your immune system. Recent research has shown that even a single seven-day course of antibiotics reduces the effectiveness of your immune system by 25%. Since antibiotics reduce the capability of your own body to combat infections, the net result is a stronger likelihood of another infection.

GLEASON SCORE EXPLAINED

The Gleason score is a measurement that is given to indicate the aggressiveness of the prostate cancer. Aggressiveness is a medical term used to describe the likelihood of the cancer spreading outside the prostate. The Gleason scoring system was developed at a VA hospital in the 1960s by Dr. Gleason and was quickly adopted all over the world as an effective predictor of the pace of prostate cancer growth.

How Does It Work?

When he created this measurement, Dr. Gleason assigned a number between 1 and 5 to the different patterns of prostate cancer cell growth. Prostate cancer cells display different patterns of growth which reveal their aggressiveness.

When your pathologist checks your biopsy samples, they examine your prostate cells under the microscope, and will look at the different patterns. They will then choose the two most commonly appearing patterns and give you a score. The first number indicates the most common pattern in all the samples. The second is the second most common pattern. When these two scores are added together, the total is called the Gleason score. This means if the two most commonly appearing patterns are Gleason 3 and Gleason 4, your cancer is primarily made up of cells that fit pattern 3 and to a lesser extent cells that match pattern 4. If this is your score, it will be written As Gleason 7 (3+4) or Gleason Score 3+4 = 7.

The order of the numbers is therefore very important, since the first score is the most common pattern of prostate cancer cells. This means that a Gleason score 4+3=7 tumour is thought to be more aggressive and fast growing than a 3+4=7 tumor.

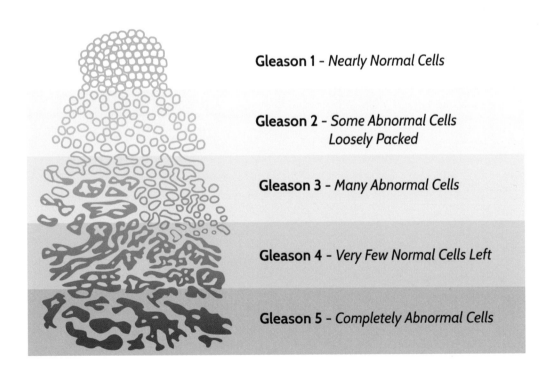

Gleason 1 - *Nearly Normal Cells*

Gleason 2 - *Some Abnormal Cells Loosely Packed*

Gleason 3 - *Many Abnormal Cells*

Gleason 4 - *Very Few Normal Cells Left*

Gleason 5 - *Completely Abnormal Cells*

It is worth noting that patterns 1 and 2 are rarely seen, either because they are hard to distinguish from healthy cells, or because biopsies are rarely conducted on men who have such low scores. Because patterns 1 and 2 are rarely seen, the lowest Gleason score of a cancer found on a prostate biopsy is 6. The highest a Gleason can be is 10.

The higher your Gleason score, the greater the likelihood of your cancer spreading outside the prostate.

Problems with Gleason score

In about 20% of cases the biopsy grade is lower than the true grade since the biopsy misses a higher grade area of the cancer. Additionally, it is also possible to overestimate the aggressiveness of a tumor as well. The other problem with Gleason score is that it requires a biopsy to be conducted. However the issues with this are all related to the biopsy itself and not the scoring system and so are addressed in that section of this report.

MAGNETIC RESONANCE IMAGING (MRI)

A Magnetic Resonance Image (MRI) body scan is often used to establish whether prostate cancer has spread (metastasized) beyond the prostate. MRIs are completely non-invasive tests, and the latest MRI technology produces very high-resolution results. This high-resolution image makes MRIs 45% more accurate than biopsies when it comes to finding aggressive cancers that have spread.

As a general rule, I advise people to avoid having too many scans since a scan exposes you to electro-magnetic radiation, which can increase cancer risk. But if you have cancer and you want to locate its' spread, an MRI is your best bet. The amount of harmful radiation from an MRI is far less than that from X-Rays. At times, the radiologist will ask for the use of dyes to gain greater contrast images. The majority of these dies are highly toxic. For example, gadolinium is a rare earth element with paramagnetic properties commonly used for MRI contrast. "Paramagnetic properties" means that the magnetic materials used for the test are weakly attracted to one another by an external magnetic field (produced by the MRI machine). These materials form internal magnetic fields in the body that linger long after the MRI test is over.

A patient will rarely see the packaging for gadolinium, which clearly shows a black box warning. Gadolinium significantly increases your risk of developing Nephrogenic Systemic Fibrosis (NSF), a kidney disorder that can lead to kidney damage requiring dialysis, and in worse possible cases, may lead to death. It is prudent, therefore, to go into MRI with caution about the use of contrast dye. And, if you are going to have an MRI, your best bet is a 3 Tesla MRI machine, which is 3 times more powerful than a traditional MRI and provides a far higher resolution, which is essential to really see what is going on.

COLOR ULTRASOUND (SONOGRAM)

Prostate ultrasound (US) tests—also referred to as sonograms—are safe, painless, and inexpensive. Unlike other screening methods, USs can be repeated as often as necessary to closely monitor areas of concern and assess treatment efficacy, and without the risk of side effects. To perform the US, the technician places a small, lubricated probe (about a finger's width) into your rectum. The US probe gives off high-frequency sound waves that you cannot hear. These sound waves enter the prostate and create echoes through the region of the pelvis. The probe then picks up the echoes, sends them back to a computer, and the computer turns them into an image that shows the prostate on the computer screen. The procedure typically takes less than 10 minutes in your doctor's office. Aside from feeling a small amount of pressure when the probe is inserted into the rectum, this procedure is not painful.

A tumor must have blood flow in order to form or exist. In many cases, altered blood flow to an area of the body can be seen years before a tumor develops. A Color Doppler Ultrasound is a specific type of US that allows the doctor to observe and measure blood flow that feeds—and always precedes—a tumor. The amount of blood flow indicates the aggressiveness of a tumor. Areas of increased blood flow are more likely to contain cancer, and a tumor without much blood flow is likely static or diminishing. Unfortunately, I am unaware of any facility in the UK, either NHS or private, that provides a Color Doppler US at the time of this writing. My Advanced Prostate Cancer Risk Assessment (APCRA, which I describe below) in Arizona does use color ultrasound, however, and to great effect.

I should caution that it is not the machine that provides the analysis. The machine only picks up and shows the image. It is up to the expertise and experience of the diagnostician to analyze the results. Also, physicians typically rely on US in combination with the results of other diagnostic tests to get a better picture of what is going on with your prostate.

4K SCORE TEST

The only test that can predict the likelihood of death from prostate cancer is the 4Kscore test. The 4Kscore uses a combination of the blood-screening tests that I discussed above—PSA and PCA3—in a comprehensive statistical analysis that compares your results with the results from men who have been diagnosed with prostate cancer over the past 20 years. You might as well ask the obvious question, which is, how can they make these comparisons since these tests did not exist 20 years ago? The answer can be found in blood banks. It is possible to do these tests retrospectively even on blood from a cancer patient who has now deceased. Blood banks provide the statistical basis for the predictions going forward from today, which makes the 4Kscore test the most accurate predictor of prostate cancer and its aggressiveness.

I do have a couple of cautions to add though. First of all, the 4Kscore should be part of a wider assessment by a highly experienced specialist physician, as we do in my clinic in Arizona. So, for example, it should be done together with a Color Doppler US in combination with an analysis of all the other data (DRE, PSA, PSA3) that is available.

The second and more important caveat is that it is important to understand that we are dealing with a statistical prediction and not a crystal-ball view about what will happen to you. The 4Kscore test provides a statistical prediction based on others. It is possible to defy the statistical odds. Certainly, taking your health into your hands and making nutrition and lifestyle changes can help!

ADVANCED PROSTATE CANCER RISK ASSESSMENT (APCRA)

The Advanced Prostate Cancer Risk Assessment (APCRA) is the most comprehensive prostate cancer diagnostic test currently available. We provide this test at my clinic in Arizona. The APCRA provides more information than a biopsy but is not invasive, and it also provides more information than an MRI, making it safer and more effective than the diagnostic tests typically relied on.

The APCRA consists of a 3 hour-consultation with a naturopathic physician who is also a professor of urology. During this extensive consultation, you will also receive a 4-dimensional Power Color Doppler Ultrasound, which is capable of much finer detection than a standard US, particularly when guided and analyzed by an expert. Many suggest that the Color Doppler scan on its own is as accurate as a biopsy, but when the results are analyzed with other tests included in the APCRA, you will have a far more detailed, informative, and accurate assessment than if you had undergone a biopsy or any of the other tests alone. The additional tests include an up-to-date PSA (including percent % of free PSA), a prostatic acid phosphatase (PAP) test, a saliva test to provide a comprehensive analysis of your available hormone balances (including testosterone, estrogen, progesterone, and others), an alkaline phosphatase test, and most importantly, a PCA3 test, which we send to independant and accredited America based urological labs.

Because the results of all those additional tests are not available at the time of your first visit, the APCRA also includes an additional diagnostic session over the telephone. This follow-up consultation takes about an hour to discuss the results of the additional tests in light of the Color Doppler US. This means you receive a preliminary diagnosis at the time of your first visit, and a more certain basis for diagnosis in the follow-up call with the additional data that comes in. The APCRA also includes a detailed, written report that can serve as a baseline for future reference, evidence for you doctor if you wish to have your prostate condition monitored "back home," or necessary information to enable you to understand your condition and the therapies to treat it.

Most importantly, the APCRA makes possible postponing a biopsy, and may even provide the necessary information to altogether forego one. It is only when you know exactly what is happening inside your prostate that you can make informed judgments about whether you should have treatment, what treatment to have, and monitor the results of any treatment you do have.

DETERMINING THE GRADE OF PROSTATE CANCER

If you have had any of the battery of tests I described above, and if your doctor suspects prostate cancer, or if you've already been diagnosed, then you may be familiar with some of the terms used to grade cancer cells or determine if a tumor has spread, and if so how much. The Gleason Score is the measure doctors use to determine how aggressive the cancer cells are. Gleason score can only be determined by getting a sample of the cells, either from biopsy or surgery. But there are other ways of staging prostate cancer, which do not require a biopsy or surgery. The TNM (Tumor-Node-Metastasis) staging system is compiled from both the DRE and other tests, like the MRI or Color Doppler scans. The TNM system tells you the size of the tumor, whether or not it has spread to lymph nodes, and if it has metastasized to other parts of the body.

The staging looks like this:

"T" indicates tumor size.

- T1: Indicates that the tumor cannot be felt on DRE or seen by the naked eye on scans.
- T2: Indicates that the tumor is confined to the prostate gland.
- T3: Indicates that the tumor has spread past the margins of the prostate gland and into the surrounding tissues.

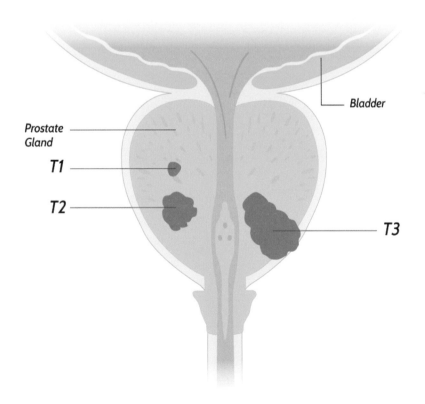

- T4: Indicates that the tumor has spread into other nearby tissues, like the rectum and bladder.

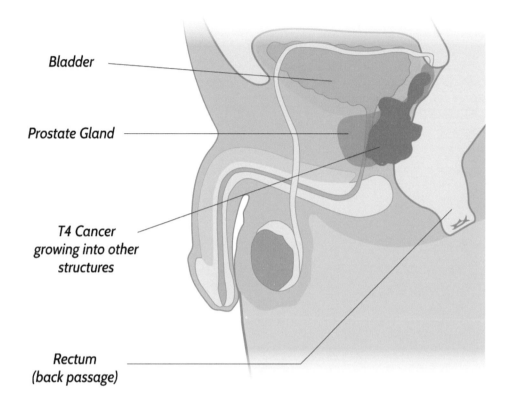

Bladder

Prostate Gland

T4 Cancer
growing into other
structures

Rectum
(back passage)

"N" indicates whether the cancer has spread to one or more lymph nodes.

- NX: Indicates that the lymph nodes have not been assessed.
- NO: Indicates that there is no sign of the tumor in nearby lymph nodes.
- N1: Indicates that a small tumor has been found in a nearby lymph node.
- N2: Indicates that a medium-sized tumor has been found in a lymph node, or several smaller tumors are seen in several lymph nodes (by MRI scan)
- N3: Indicates that a large tumor has been found in one or more lymph nodes.

"M" indicates that the cancer has spread past the lymph nodes.

- MX: Indicates that it is not known if the cancer has spread to other tissues in the body.
- MO: Indicates that the cancer has not spread to other locations.
- M1a: Indicates that cancer has spread to distant lymph nodes
- M1b: Indicates that cancer has spread into the bones
- M1c: Indicates that cancer has spread into other distant tissues or organs in the body.

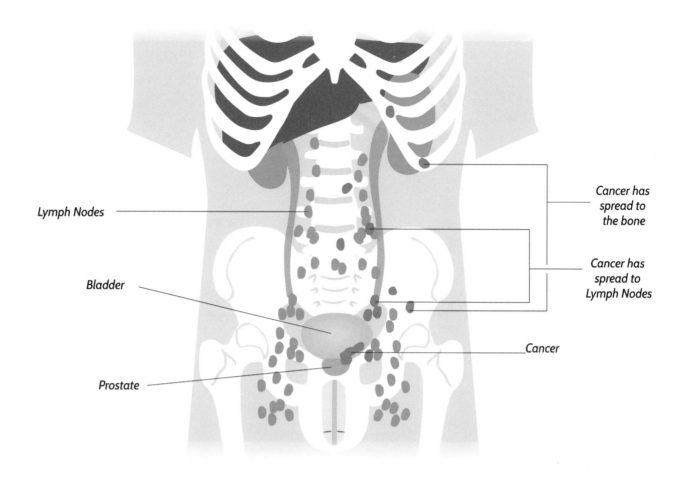

Lymph Nodes

Bladder

Prostate

Cancer has spread to the bone

Cancer has spread to Lymph Nodes

Cancer

PROSTATE CANCER STAGES

Stage	Stage Grouping	Stage Description
I	T1, N0, M0 Gleason score 6 or less PSA less than 10	The doctor can't feel the tumor or see it with an imaing test such as transrectal ultrasound (it was either found during a transurethal resection or it was diagnosed by needle biopsy done for a high PSA) [T1]. The cancer is still within the prostate and has not spread to nearby lymph nodes [N0] or elsewhere in the body [M0]. The Gleason score is 6 or less and the PSA level is less than 10.

Stage	Stage Grouping	Stage Description
I	OR	
	T2a, N0, M0 Gleason score 6 or less PSA less than 10	The tumour can be felt by digital rectal exam or seen with imaging such as transrectal ultrasound and is in one half or less of only one side (left or right) of the prostate [T2a]. The cancer is still within the prostate and has not spread to nearby lymph nodes [N0] or elsewhere in the body [M0]. The Gleason score is 6 ot less and the PSA level is less than 10.
2A	T1, N0, M0 Gleason score 7 PSA less than 20	The doctor can't feel the tumor or see it with imaging such as transrectal ultrasound (it was either found during a transurethral resection or was diagnosed by needle biopsy done for a high PSA level) [T1]. The cancer has not spread to nearby lymph nodes [N0] or elsewhere in the body [M0]. The tumor has a Gleason score of 7. The PSA level is less than 20.
	OR	
	T1, N0, M0 Gleason score 6 or less PSA at least 10 but less than 20	The doctor can't feel the tumor or see it with imaging such as transrectal ultrasound (it was either found during a transurethral resection or was diagnosed by needle biopsy done for a high PSA) [T1]. The cancer has not spread to nearby lymph nodes [N0] or elsewhere in the body [M0]. The tumorn has a Gleason score of 6 or less. The PSA level is at least 10 but less than 20.

Stage	Stage Grouping	Stage Description
2A	**OR**	
	2a or T2b, N0, M0 Gleason score of 7 or less PSA less than 20	The tumor can be felt by digital rectal exam or seen with imaging such as transrectal ultrasound and is in only one side of the prostate [T2a or T2b]. The cancer has not spread to nearby lymph node [N0] or elsewhere in the body [M0]. It has a Gleason score of 7 or less. The PSA level is less than 20.
2B	T2c, N0, M0 Any Gleason score Any PSA	The tumor can be felt by digital rectal exam or seen with imaging such as transrectal ultrasound and is in both sides of the prostate [T2c]. The cancer has not spread to nearby lymph nodes [N0] or elsewhere in the body [M0]. The tumor can have any gleason score and the PSA can be any value.
	OR	
	T1 or T2, N0, M0 Any Gleason score PSA of 20 or more	The cancer has not yet spread outside the prostate. It may (or may not) be felt by digital rectal exam or seen with imaging such as trans-rectal ultrasound [T1 or T2]. The cancer has not spread to nearby lymph nodes [N0] or elsewhere in the body [M0]. The tumor can have any Gleason score. The PSA level is at least 20.
	OR	

Stage	Stage Grouping	Stage Description
2B	T1 or T2, N0, M0 Gleason score of 8 or higher Any PSA	The cancer has not yet spread outside the prostate. It may (or may not) be felt by digital rectal exam or seen with imaging such as transrectal ultrasound [T1 or T2]. The cancer has not spread to nearby lymph nodes [N0] or elsewhere in the body [M0]. The Gleason score is 8 or higher. The PSA can be any value.
3	T2c, N0, M0 Any Gleason score Any PSA	The cancer has grown outside the prostate and may have spread to the seminal vesicles [T3], but ithas not spread to nearby lymph nodes [N0] or elsewhere in the body [M0]. The Gleason scroe is 8 or higher. The PSA can be any value.
4	T4, N0, M0 Any Gleason score Any PSA	The cancer has grown into tissues next to the prostate (other than the seminal vesicles), such as the urethral sphincter (muscle that helps control urination), rectum, bladder, and/or the wall of the pelvis [T4]. The cancer has not spread to nearby lymph nodes [N0] or elsewhere in the body [M0]. The tumor can have any Gleason score and the PSA can be any value.
	OR	

Stage	Stage Grouping	Stage Description
4	Any T, N1, M0 Any Gleason score Any PSA	The tumor may or may not be growing into tissues near the prostate [any T]. The cancer has spread to nearby lymph nodes [N1] but has not spread elsewhere in the body [M0]. The tumor can have any Gleason score and the PSA can be any value.
	OR	
	Any T, any N, M1 Any Gleason score Any PSA	The cancer may or may not be growing into tissues near the prostate [any T] and may or may not have spread to nearby lymph nodes [any N]. It has spread to other, more distant sites in the body [M1]. The tumor can have any Gleason score and the PSA can be any value.

*Table sourced from the American Cancer Society

CONVENTIONAL MEDICAL TREATMENT FOR BPH

I discussed above that most physicians still operate under the notion that too much testosterone causes prostate disease. If this idea is what your doctor believes, then the likely starting point for treating you will be trying to radically lower your testosterone levels, and if this doesn't counter your prostate disease, and it likely won't, then your physician will try more invasive measure and eventually remove your prostate tissue altogether. This approach doesn't get at the underlying problem of what causes prostate disease in the first place, which I will discuss in Part 2. In this section, however, I want to provide a list of the treatments that might be presented to you if you are diagnosed with BPH or prostate cancer.

CONVENTIONAL MEDICAL TREATMENT FOR BPH

Here are the treatments that medical doctors use to treat BPH, starting with the least invasive, which is hormone therapy, and moving along to the more invasive approaches.

Hormone Therapy

There are two drugs approved by the FDA and proscribed for an enlarged prostate. A word of caution before moving on to the discussion about these drugs, it is my opinion and that of many others that approval by the FDA does not mean a drug is safe. The majority of drugs cause side effects, some of them life-threatening, and these side effects often need to be treated by ... other drugs! Drug therapies can start a cycle of snowball effects, and it is always wise to proceed with caution when considering taking any pharmaceuticals—even those that are "over-the-counter."

5-alpha-Reductase Inhibitors

The most widely used drug for the treatment of BPH is finasteride, sold under the brand name of Proscar®. Finasteride is a 5-alpha-reductase inhibitor, meaning it prevents the enzyme 5 alpha-reductase from converting testosterone into DHT. You will recall that DHT causes growth of the prostate, so Proscar® is designed to shrink the enlarged prostate gland by reducing the amount of DHT in the bloodstream. There are two types of 5 alpha-reductase. Type 1 is present in tissues outside the prostate gland, such as liver or skin, and type 2 is found predominantly in the prostate. Finasteride acts as an inhibitor of type 2 5α-reductase enzyme.

Studies have shown that finasteride reduces intraprostatic DHT levels by 91.4%. This information has raised concerns by some researchers and physicians, and patients alike, for fear that the drug reduces DHT levels so much as to chemically castrate a man. This is not so, however, because finasteride does not act on Type 1 5 alpha-reductase. There is still enough circulating testosterone to be converted to DHT by the type 1 isoenzyme found in the skin and liver.

By lowering DHT levels, finasteride decreases the size of the prostate. This process takes between 3 and 6 months before the clinical effects kick in and the prostate reduces in size. Therefore, the efficacy of finasteride cannot be felt until a patient has been on the medication for a while. But side effects from the drug can begin to manifest in a matter of days or weeks and can get worse over time.

Safety of Finasteride (and other 5-alpha-Reductase Inhibitors)

A number of side effects have been reported with the use of finasteride and other 5 alpha-reductase inhibitors. In referring below to finasteride, I am referring also to the other 5- alpha-reductase inhibitors as well. A placebo-controlled study of 1,524 patients treated with finasteride and 1516 patients treated with placebo were followed over a period of 4 years.

The most frequently reported adverse reactions were related to sexual function.

- 8.1 % of men reported regular impotence
- 6.4 % of men reported decreased libido
- 3.7% of men saw a decreased volume of ejaculate

Less common side effects include the growth of male breasts; tenderness, soreness and pain in male breasts; rashes, allergic reactions, itching, hives, and swelling of the lips and face.
Some men reported testicular pain, and there was a weak link to increased risk of developing male breast cancer. Another concern that has been pointed out is that finasteride may mask the signs of aggressive—yet curable if caught early enough—prostate cancers until later in their growth, which may make them more lethal.

Other studies have since reported that finasteride may reduce the incidence of prostate cancer, although these are controversial results. It appears that finasteride may lower your risk of slow-growing prostate cancers while increasing your risk of aggressive prostate cancer. The largest study investigating prostate cancer prevention with Finasteride was published in 2003. The researchers noted a 24.8% risk reduction in the prevalence of prostate cancer over seven years between the finasteride group and the placebo group. However, they also noted an alarming increase in high-grade tumors (Gleason Score of 7 or above) in the finasteride group (37%) when compared to the placebo group (22%).

New research also shows that some men experience cognitive effects from taking finasteride. These cognitive side effects, in conjunction with the sexual side effects, can persist for as long as 10 years after men stop taking the drug. A 2014 meta-study coined the phrase *post-finasteride syndrome* and noted that "Many clinicians are unaware of the scope of the persistent physical and psychological adverse effects of finasteride. Symptoms range from minor to severe." Other studies report similar conclusions.

Efficacy of Finasteride (and other 5-alpha-Reductase Inhibitors)

Studies show that finasteride does reduce symptoms related to prostate enlargement and that it is effective at reducing the size of the prostate. Just after it was approved by the FDA, a large-scale study was conducted examining the efficacy of finasteride. In this study, 895 subjects with BPH were randomized to receive a placebo, 1mg, or 5 mg of finasteride over a period of 1 year. The primary outcome measures consisted of a symptom score and a peak flow rate. Measurements of prostate size were also recorded. The symptom score measures the total scores of nine symptoms, including decreased urinary stream, dribbling, interruption in the stream, hesitancy, feeling of incomplete emptying, straining to initiate flow, urgency, incontinence, and dysuria. The group taking the normal 5 mg oral dose of finasteride per day showed a statistical improvement in symptoms (21% improvement) compared with the placebo group (just 2%). Another group taking a lower dose of finasteride (1mg oral per day) saw no statistical improvement in symptoms over the placebo group.

Studies have demonstrated that this reduction in urinary symptoms is associated with prostate size at the beginning of the treatment. In other words, the smaller the prostate at onset of treatment, the less the symptomatic relief. Men with more enlarged prostates (>25 ml) at onset of treatment tend to have the most significant reduction in symptoms. In general, finasteride seems to cause a modest improvement in BPH symptoms after a 12-month period.

Finasteride does shrink the prostate and therefore appears to have some benefit. But, as I indicated above, the greatest benefit seems to occur for men with larger prostates at onset of treatment. Studies have shown that the reduction in prostate size is sustained for 5 years following a 1 year course of finasteride treatment. They also note that the majority of the benefits and effects of finasteride on prostate size will be achieved within 6 months.

Concluding Remarks on Finasteride

Men's responses to finasteride vary widely, both in its efficacy and side effects. Your response to the drug will be highly individualized and unique to you. It is a good idea to consider the following factors when deciding whether or not to take finasteride: first, prostate size. We can see from the studies I reported above that the largest indicator of efficacy is the size of the prostate at the onset of treatment. Second, it will behove you to consider whether or not you can or want to wait 6–12 months for an average 20% reduction in symptoms. Third, weighing in on the cancer risks is important: the decreased risk of less aggressive cancers to the increased risk of more aggressive cancers. Fourth, there are the cognitive and psychological side effects to bear in mind. Fifth, the significance of the sexual side effects is important to factor in. Based on feedback from our clinical and customer-service teams, the primary complaint and regret from men who take finasteride is the sexual side effects. Sixth, there are the infrequently discussed concerns about the effects of this drug on pregnant women who come in contact with the it or the sperm of a man who has taken finasteride. And finally, finasteride can also lower a man's PSA levels by as much as 60%. This lower PSA level is very important to note, because a falsely low PSA level can interfere with detecting prostate cancer.

Also, not all BPH problems come from expansion of glandular tissue. For some men, the prostate gland is normal in size, but because the smooth-muscle tissue in the prostate has begun to contract around the urethra, these men also suffer from painful BPH symptoms. There is an additional drug for this set of problems (see next section).

Alpha Blockers

Another category of drugs, called alpha blockers, is prescribed for BPH symptoms. Alpha-blockers, like terazosin (the generic version), marketed under the product names Hytrin®, or tamsulosin, under the name, Flomax®, relax the smooth muscle of the prostate gland and neck of the bladder to improve urine flow. In the late 1970s, an alpha-blocker named phenoxybenzamine was shown to be effective in treating the symptoms of BPH. The problem with this drug was that about 30% of patients experienced serious side effects. It was later identified as being a potentially strong carcinogen. Tamsulosin became available in 1996 and was promoted as a breakthrough because men suffered fewer side effects than phenoxybenzamine. Tamsulosin (Flomax®) is now the most commonly prescribed drug for men with symptoms of BPH.

Alpha blockers work by binding to alpha-adrenergic receptors, preventing the receptor from being stimulated. Alpha-adrenergic receptors are stimulated by stress hormones, such as epinephrine. The effect is to shuttle blood flow toward skeletal muscle and away from what the body deems "non-essential" functions during stress or physical demand. Alpha blockers, therefore, inhibit this process and allow for the smooth muscles in the body to relax, such as those around the prostate, in the bladder, urethra, and blood vessels. As a result, urine flows more freely.

Safety of Alpha Blockers

For men complaining of urgency, the need to urinate frequently, or difficulty completely emptying the bladder, alpha blockers might be prescribed. These drugs not only relax the smooth muscles around the prostate and bladder but also the smooth muscles throughout the body, such as veins and arteries. So, unfortunately, alpha blockers can also have undesirable side effects, including headaches, fatigue, nasal congestion, dizziness, and syncope (fainting).

A big cause for concern is severe hypotension (low blood pressure) because alpha blockers relax the smooth muscles in the heart, just as they do in other places in the body. The result is that the heart is less effective at pumping blood to the rest of the body, including the brain. Also, because blood vessels throughout the body are relaxed, veins are less effective at getting blood back to the heart. A cohort study involving 14,784 men compared those who used an alpha blocker from 2003 to 2013 with an equal number of men who did not in order to examine whether alpha blockers increased the risk of falling due to hypotension. Those who used of alpha-blockers experienced an increased risk of falling by 14% compared to men who did not use alpha blockers. Also, alpha blockers have been shown to cause complications during cataract surgery and result in floppy eye syndrome.

Studies show that men often discontinue use of alpha blockers due to the intensity of side effects. A Cochrane systematic review looked at the effects of tamsulosin for BPH. While the study participants did report improvements in symptoms, they also consistently reported experiencing dizziness, rhinitis (runny nose), and abnormal ejaculation compared to those in the study who took a placebo. Side effects are worse with higher doses, and many men experience sexual dysfunction, including ED, retrograde ejaculation, and decreased libido.

Efficacy of Alpha Blockers

Evidence suggests that alpha blockers are moderately effective at best in reducing symptoms, which are not likely to go away completely when taking these medications. As with finasteride, the size of the prostate determines the effectiveness of alpha blockers. They are notably less effective when the prostate is larger. Because they do not act on the prostate gland itself—only the smooth muscles and blood vessels around it—alpha-blockers do not slow down the growth of the prostate. A 2008 study found that prostate size did not change, and PSA levels increased by 12.1% over two years of tamsulosin use. Alpha blockers, therefore, will also not reduce the risk of developing prostate cancer.

Concluding Remarks on Alpha Blockers

The vast majority of industry-funded studies on BPH-specific alpha blockers, (i.e., tamsulosin) remain unpublished. Independent studies raise questions about the efficacy and safety of this medication. Its high rate of side effects and low efficacy means patients may wish to consider alternative treatments.

Alpha blockers do not cure BPH. The prostate continues to enlarge, and over time, higher doses of the medication are necessary to treat the urinary symptoms. Eventually, surgery will be necessary if there are no other therapies to address the fact that the prostate is enlarging. Also, muscles that are relaxed by these drugs can fall into disuse and weaken, increasing the chances of incontinence later on.

Surgery

As I offered earlier, another approach to the treatment of benign prostate disease is to remove the prostate gland altogether. There are a couple of ways that urologists might go about doing so surgically.

Transurethral Resection of the Prostate (TURP)

Transurethral Resection of the Prostate (TURP) is a surgical procedure that doesn't require external incision. Most doctors suggest using TURP instead of making an incision into the body to access the prostate, and at least 90 % of all prostate surgeries for BPH are TURP. With a TURP, an instrument called a resectoscope is inserted through the penis to get to the prostate gland. The resectoscope, which is about 12 inches long and 1/2 inch in diameter, consists of a light, valves for controlling fluid that is used to irrigate the area, and an electrical loop that cuts tissue and seals off the blood vessels.

During this 90-minute operation, the surgeon uses the resectoscope's wire loop to chisel away at the prostate tissue one little piece at a time. The pieces of tissue are carried by the fluid into the bladder and then flushed out of the body at the end of the operation.

Because they do not require an incision to access the prostate, TURPs are less traumatic than open forms of surgery and require a shorter recovery period. They do, however, require anesthesia and an overnight stay in the hospital. There are also possible side effects, like retrograde (backward) ejaculation. In this condition, semen flows back into the bladder during climax instead of out the urethra.

Transurethral Incision of the Prostate (TUIP)

Another surgical procedure used for BPH is called transurethral incision of the prostate (TUIP). Instead of removing prostate tissue, as with the TURP, this procedure widens the urethra by making a few small cuts in the neck of the bladder and in the prostate gland. The "neck" is where the urethra joins the bladder.

Although some people believe that TUIP gives the same relief as TURP with fewer side effects, the truth is that there is not enough information yet about the real advantages and side effects of this procedure. I cannot overemphasize that with all surgical procedures, there is some risk. In addition, with the TUIP, as with the alpha blockers, the prostate will continue to grow, and typically, within two years or more, the problems can reoccur.

Laser Surgeries

In March 1996, the FDA approved a surgical procedure that uses lasers to treat the prostate. These are side-firing laser fibers and Nd:YAG lasers that vaporize obstructing prostate tissue. During the laser procedure, the doctor passes the laser fiber into the penis and through the urethra to get to the area near the prostate. The device they use to pass the laser through the urethra is called a cystoscope. Once the end of the cystoscope is in place, the urologist signals the laser to deliver several bursts of laser energy that last anywhere from 30 to 60 seconds. The laser energy destroys prostate tissue, causing the prostate gland to shrink. As with a TURP, laser surgery requires anesthesia and a stay in the hospital.

One advantage of laser surgery over TURP is that laser surgery causes very little blood loss and allows for a quicker recovery time. But laser surgery may not be effective on prostates that are particularly enlarged. Also, the long-term effectiveness of laser surgery is not yet known.

There are newer procedures available that use laser technology and can be performed on an outpatient basis. Photoselective Vaporization of the Prostate (PVP) is one such procedure. PVP uses a high-energy laser that is absorbed by aspects of the blood (hemoglobin) but not by water. When PVP is applied to the prostate, the laser light becomes absorbed by the blood in the vascularized prostate tissue, which vaporizes it and seals the treated area. This creates a "prostate cavity" with very little blood loss. Interstitial Laser Coagulation (ILC) places the tip of the laser fiber optic probe directly into the prostate tissue and fires the laser to destroy it.

CONVENTIONAL MEDICAL TREATMENT FOR PROSTATE CANCER

Let's be honest, a cancer diagnosis is scary. Any time we hear the "C" word, we startle into the fear of dying. Now, with a diagnosis like prostate cancer, I think it's safe to say that the medical establishment is, in large measure, responsible for this anxiety, because a prostate cancer diagnosis is not necessarily a death sentence, as I discussed earlier. In early stage prostate cancer, and by this I mean localized, non-aggressive prostate cancer, the diagnosis is arguably more damaging than the cancer itself. The idea that we have cancer hurls us immediately into the intense desire to get rid of it—as quickly as possible.

Physicians respond with a whole plethora of treatments aimed at eradicating the cancer.
But eradicating cancer also means eradicating parts of our body. In a very high percentage of cases, leaving localized prostate cancer alone is more called for than removing it. The same is not true for aggressive, metastasizing prostate cancer. Of all men combined, the rate of "latent" cancer or cancer found at autopsy is much greater than the rate of clinical cancer, possibly as high as 80% by age 80 years. In other words, lots of men die with undetected prostate cancer from causes unrelated to prostate cancer.

Bear with me while I jump on a little soap box of concern that I have about early detection and treatment. When mainstream medicine points to a lower mortality rate now than in previous decades for prostate cancer, they suggest that early detection and more sophisticated treatment methods are reducing prostate-cancer-related deaths. I believe this analysis is self-serving. Certainly, detection is earlier. But is conventional prostate-cancer treatment any more effective than it was previously? I'm not convinced that it is. My concern is that early detection is roping in people whose prostate cancers are so slight that these early detection efforts increase the number of people diagnosed and treated but who would never have known otherwise that they have prostate cancer, nor would they die of it no matter what treatment they did or did not receive. In other words, these analyses about early detection and lower mortality rates strike me as a statistical quirk that has no real meaning. Of course, every person has to choose where he falls along the spectrum of belief.

Certainly, there is considerable evidence that conventional treatments for prostate cancer cause substantial damage to the quality-of-life for those patients receiving these treatments. While new technologies like laser surgery can reduce some of the collateral damage seen in the older open surgery techniques, there remains considerable potential for long-term problems, even with these new technologies. When we look back at medical practices in general, even those practiced not very long ago, we are starting to recognize that some of those treatments were brutal, ignorant, and completely misguided. I mentioned a few such practices earlier in this guide and how long it took for important changes to happen. There are many more such scenarios.

Conventional medicine, like all science and technology, is always changing, not only its understandings about diseases, but with that, its treatment methods. Medical perspectives on diseases go hand-in-hand with treatment practices. It is my opinion that in twenty or thirty years' time, the consensus will view much of the current outlook on localized prostate cancer and treatment as misguided.

Great progress could be made by conventional medicine if only it would start treating the research on cause (including diet!) with the respect it deserves. This means taking the underlying root of the problem into account. It also means seeking to remedy that rather than simply attacking symptoms.

All Conventional Medical Therapies for Prostate Cancer Have Serious Side Effects

It is not an accident that there is a great deal of confusion about the different types of prostate cancer treatments and their side effects. Let's look for a moment at a typical treatment scenario. If a hospital specializes in one form of prostate cancer therapy, the research and analysis from this hospital will almost certainly be skewed to show that this particular therapy is more effective than other therapies. This is not always the case, but most certainly, it is the typical scenario. The hospital markets this information for both reputation and financial reasons. And prostate cancer is big business. So, it can be quite a daunting task as a healthcare consumer to get at the truth of efficacy and/or potential damage(s) associated with any therapy.

The reality is that any treatment that destroys tissue is likely to have side effects. It doesn't matter whether you cut it out with a knife, burn it out with a laser, freeze it out, or irradiate it to death. The bottom line is that all treatments that destroy tissue take away what has evolved over eons to perform a function. It's simple, when you destroy the tissue, you also destroy its function. And that loss of function almost inevitably has ripple effects that affect quality-of-life. Nature didn't put tissues in the body that are not necessary.

A 2002 report published in the Journal of Clinical Oncology compared the quality-of-life between men who received no treatment (controls) and those who received one of several different prostate cancer treatments for localized prostate cancer (meaning, non-aggressive, no metastases). These options included brachytherapy (radioactive "seeds" placed inside the prostate), standard "external-beam" radiation, and surgery. Brachytherapy, as we shall see below, is intended to have fewer side effects because the radiation is placed in the local area of the prostate rather than being "beamed" from the outside and across a number of other tissues that are then in "caught in the line of fire."

In the study, 1,014 men treated for localized prostate cancer at the University of Michigan between the years of 1995–1999 replied to questionnaires at an average of two years after treatment about how bothered they were by any sexual, urinary, or bowel problems. The study found that sexual function was "a big or moderate problem" reported by 60% of the men treated with brachytherapy, 46% of those treated with external-beam radiation, and 50% of those treated with surgery. These men also reported that urinary function was "a big or moderate problem" by about 27% of those treated with brachytherapy, about 10% of those treated with external-beam radiation, and about 8% of those treated with surgery. There were similar concerns about bowel problems. Difficulties with bowel function were felt to be "a big or moderate problem" by 17% of those treated with brachytherapy, 7% of those treated with external beam radiation, and 3% of those treated surgically. In other words, sexual and urinary and bowel problems bothered more brachytherapy patients than external radiation treatment or surgery, and those receiving no treatment at all reported fewer problems than any among the treatment groups. Yet, brachytherapy is supposed to be a better, more localized treatment option with fewer side effects than external beam radiation.

The report concluded that overall health-related quality-of-life was compromised for all patients treated with conventional methods when compared to those who received no treatment. "There are different types of side effects typical of those different therapies, but overall, the quality-of-life after treatment is not superior in any one of the three treatments," wrote study co-author Martin G. Sanda, MD, Associate Professor in the departments of Internal Medicine, Urology, and Surgery at the University of Michigan. Sanda and his colleagues noted that quality-of-life concerns, such as urinary incontinence, reduced sexual function, or bowel problems are very important to men considering prostate-cancer treatment.

Before you consider any sort of treatment, it is crucial to have a firm diagnosis that confirms the presence of prostate cancer. More importantly, it is critical to have a solid idea about whether that cancer is aggressive and likely to become life-threatening. Localized prostate cancer with a low Gleason Score is not aggressive cancer.

As I have already indicated above, I'm not a proponent of the conventional medical therapies for localized prostate cancer and a Gleason score of 7 or lower, since it is not an aggressive form of cancer. I do go over all these treatments here so that you can make informed decisions that feel right for you. Hurried doctors may not have the time to explain all that you need to know, and many, in favor of one procedure or another, will simply tell you that you need the procedure and then proceed to schedule it.

If you have a Gleason score of 9 or higher, there is a strong argument for undergoing one or more of the conventional treatments I outline here, and your urologist is likely to recommend any one or more of them. This is particularly true for men 65 and younger. The younger you are with aggressive prostate cancer, the more likely it is that your prostate cancer will become life-threatening. No matter what, I recommend making changes to your diet and lifestyle and taking supplements to boost the immune system. Natural, integrative and holistic treatments take time. With a Gleason score of 7 or more, you do not have the liberty of time to pursue only natural approaches. With a Gleason score of 6 or 7, you are much more likely to have the time that it takes for integrated treatments to take effect.

Whatever treatment you decide, if you can add additional holistic and integrative treatments, by all means do so. And at the very least, you should make the changes to your diet and lifestyle that I recommend in Part 2, and add natural supplements, which I outline in Part 3. For now, though, let's consider the conventional treatment approaches for prostate cancer—both localized and aggressive, spreading cancer.

Watchful Waiting

Many men choose watchful waiting as a rational treatment option for low-grade, localized prostate cancer. During the watchful waiting period, the physician keeps the cancer under close watch, which is why watchful waiting is also sometimes is referred to as active surveillance.

During watchful waiting, no medical treatment is provided—meaning, medications, radiation, and surgery aren't used. That means that you avoid the risks and side effects associated with those treatment options. This does not mean, however, that you shouldn't take advantage of the benefits of natural approaches in the meantime!

Watchful waiting may be recommended if your cancer isn't causing signs and symptoms, is expected to grow very slowly, and is small and localized to one area of your prostate. Many older men may live out their normal life-span without treatment and without a non-invasive prostate cancer spreading or causing other problems. Watchful waiting can also be a rational option if you're a younger man—as long as you know the facts and are willing to be vigilant about follow-up checkups. In my view, the best thing about watchful waiting is avoiding the complications and side effects from conventional treatments. But watchful waiting is a missed opportunity unless you make changes to diet and lifestyle that I recommend later in this guide.

In a Swedish ten-year study, researchers used a questionnaire was to record symptoms of sexual, urinary, and bowel function, along with some quality-of-life indicators, during the first four years after surgery or with watchful waiting instead. For sexual function, 80% of men in the surgery group had difficulty obtaining an erection compared with 45% in the watchful waiting group. 'Distress' due to impaired sexual function was reported as moderate or great in 56% of the men who had surgery and in 40% of the watchful-waiting men.

Urinary leaking was more common after surgery than with watchful waiting—49% versus 21%, respectfully. On the other hand, symptoms of urinary obstruction (difficulty starting urine, slow stream, or a feeling of not completely emptying the bladder) were more frequent in the watchful-waiting group. A weak stream was reported by 44% of these men compared with 28% in the surgery group. The side effects of each approach were clearly different with respect to sexual and urinary function. Across the board, however, disturbances of sexual function, bowel function, anxiety, depression, and well-being were more marked in the group that had treatments.

Hormone Therapy

I place hormone therapy here because it is a first line of defense, often used in combination with external radiation therapy. The same hormone therapies used for BPH are used for prostate cancer. Please refer to the section above for a review of hormone therapy.

External Radiation Treatment

The most common prostate cancer treatment is radiation therapy (XRT), and particularly its oldest form, electron-beam radiation therapy. Doctors typically recommend XRT when the prostate tumor has spread beyond the outer limits of the prostate and into to surrounding tissues, which would correspond with a tumor grade of T3 to T4. The radiation destroys cancer cells and shrinks tumors. The main advantage claimed for external radiation therapy is that it prevents the need for prostate-removal surgery (prostatectomy), which, as a more invasive procedure, has a higher rate of serious side effects. There is evidence that XRT is markedly less effective on obese patients.

XRT may also be used for pain relief with prostate cancer that has spread to the bones or that is no longer responding to hormone therapy. XRT has been shown to extend life in more aggressive forms of prostate cancer. A study of 999 patients found 79% of stage T1, 66% of stage T2, 55% of stage T3, and 22% of stage T4 prostate cancer patients survived 10 years after XRT.

There are newer versions of external radiation therapies, such as intensity modulated, 3D-CRT, and proton beam therapy. Whether or not these treatments are more effective and/or produce fewer side effects is yet to be determined. As I have indicated, there is a strong tendency for hospitals to offer the latest (and most expensive) therapies as marketing for their hospital.

Recently, CyberKnife® stereotactic radiosurgery has been added at some medical centers to treat prostate cancer. In this procedure, a computer program is used to determine the precise shape, size, and location of the tumor, and a robotic arm helps deliver highly concentrated beams of radiation from many different angles and positions. These beams intersect at the tumor and thus, should not damage healthy tissue.

Regardless of the type, XRT can cause a variety of side effects. Some go away after therapy stops. These side effects include tiredness, skin reactions in the treated areas, sometimes skin cancer, frequent and painful urination, upset stomach, diarrhea, and rectal irritation or bleeding. The immune system is also affected, and recovering immune health can take considerable time. Therefore, the person who has undergone XRT is at a higher risk of getting sick from viruses, bacterial infections, and so on.

There are some permanent side effects also. Bowel function may not return to normal even after treatment is complete. Many men become impotent up to two years later, which can be permanent. This is especially important for the younger patient to consider when thinking about different treatment options. There can be scarring from radiation burns that cause permanent internal pain. And surgical removal of the prostate is complicated after XRT, but if radiation fails, surgery is the next line of treatment.

Brachytherapy

Brachytherapy is a procedure in which radioactive material sealed in needles, seeds, wires, or catheters is placed directly into or near a tumor. Brachytherapy is also called internal radiation, implant radiation, and interstitial radiation. It is often used to treat early localized prostate cancer, with the aim of curing it. For this reason, one would expect high survival rates, but figures for disease-free survival after treatment vary enormously.

There are a variety of ways that doctors use brachytherapy. Some doctors mix it with external radiation. Some use low dose and others high dose variants. Some plant the seeds at the out borders of the prostate (where cancer tends to occur). Others plant them uniformly across the prostate.

Although brachytherapy should produce fewer side effects than external beam radiation (since the treatment is more localized), the Michigan study that I mentioned at the beginning of this section showed that this may not be the case. Durado Brooks, MD, Director of Prostate and Colorectal Cancer Program for the American Cancer Society noted, "This [Michigan study] was a very important and useful study because before this we didn't really have a direct, head-to-head comparison of brachytherapy with the other therapies, and yet brachytherapy has been touted as having fewer side effects." He added that "the claim that brachytherapy has fewer side effects may not be entirely true. . ." But Brooks said it's not entirely certain whether the study's conclusions can be applied to all patients with localized prostate cancer, for several reasons. For example, all the study patients were treated at The University of Michigan, whose doctors perform so many prostate operations every year that their practice at this procedure may produce better outcomes than in smaller hospitals. And since the 1995 study, the University of Michigan external-beam radiologists have started using tightly focused 3D conformal radiation, in which healthy tissue is more likely to be spared. This 3D conformal radiation technology is not available everywhere, so patients treated at other facilities may have more or different side effects.

Surgery: Radical Prostatectomy

Radical prostatectomy is an operation performed to remove the entire prostate and is only done for cancer that is thought not to have spread beyond the prostate (organ-confined). It is a major operation, which is technically demanding, and surgeons require considerable training before having the necessary skills to perform radical prostatectomies safely and effectively, causing as little damage as possible to nerves in the pelvic floor and around the penis.

There are various techniques for doing a radical prostatectomy, but an increasingly popular method is a called the keyhole technique using a laparoscope. During the keyhole technique, the surgeon makes 5 tiny incisions into the abdomen and inserts a scope into the tissue through which he or she then performs removes the prostate tissue. It takes longer to perform and is technically more demanding than a standard, open procedure. A robot can be used to help operate the instruments, which can make the operation technically easier for surgeons to learn if they don't possess the necessary laparoscopic skills.

From the patients' point of view, the laparoscopic method causes less pain afterward. It also results in less blood loss and cuts down on the need for hospitalization and catheterization. Recovery time is much shorter, therefore, than with a standard open procedure. The laparosopic method is still major surgery though, and as a result, you can anticipate side effects. The Krongrad Institute in Florida, which does nothing but laparoscopic radical prostatectomies, states on their website, "Consider radical prostatectomy an operation associated with risk of bleeding, pain, impotence, incontinence, long recovery, heart attack, clots, stroke, infection, injury, scarring and failure to cure. There is risk, discomfort and inconvenience with every prostate cancer treatment."

Prostatectomy often leads to incontinence (urinary leaking) lasting up to 18 months after surgery and then, after it does go away, the leaking often returns later on. About 40% of men have at least occasional urinary leaking after prostatectomy. Men are far more likely to be impotent after surgery because damage to nerves is common. A majority of men (60%) will be impotent 18 months after radical prostatectomy. And the majority of men experience reduced sensation of the penis.

Newer Treatments

The only new approaches to prostate cancer are to use new technologies to pursue the same long trodden paths. Cryosurgery is a new technology; the surgeon freezes tissue to destroy it. Laser approaches are still fairly new and favored by many urologists. There are also experimental methods using ultrasound and photodynamic (light) therapy to destroy tissue. One can argue for the relative merits of different technologies in terms of their accuracy and reduced collateral damage and side effects. The reality is, however, that in the last thirty years there has been no really new thinking about effective ways to treat prostate cancer. The approach remains to be what it always was: destroy tissue and eradicate hormones.

Ironically, the only new thinking is the reappearance of ancient arts of healing. Max Gerson initiated this movement. A German Jewish doctor who came to US as a refugee, Gerson worked his whole life to cure cancer with pure nutrition and natural non-invasive means. Dr. Albert Schweitzer once stated: "Max Gerson is the most eminent genius in medical history." Unfortunately, the mainstream medical establishment in the US eventually froze him out, and no one would publish his papers. His grand-daughter operates his clinic now in Mexico with some success. In Japan, two hospitals have adopted Gerson's methods in the last fifteen years with—they claim—great success. Remarkably, around the turn of this century, a highly eminent surgeon cured himself of pancreatic cancer that had metastasized to his liver, using the Gerson approach. He knew better than anyone else that his condition was incurable by his own mainstream chemotherapy and surgery treatment. He then set about treating his patients the same way. According to his statement in a documentary entitled, 'Dying to Have Known', this surgeon's clinic has treated five hundred patients with terminal cancers of all kinds with a better than 50% completely cure rate. He claims to have all the documentary evidence, but the establishment of US and European mainstream medicine will not even examine his results. His claims are noteworthy enough to consider, nevertheless, and they provide sufficient evidence for us to pay close attention to the impact of diet and lifestyle on prostate disease and cancer.

PART 2:

Natural Approaches To Health & Prostate Disease

See p9 18

NATURAL APPROACHES

Prostate disease is one of many chronic, progressive diseases. Research is telling us that the epidemic of chronic diseases is linked to our modern lifestyle, which means, by changing how we live, these diseases are not inevitable! Unlike breaking a leg, which happens suddenly, chronic diseases take quite a while to develop. We don't wake up one morning and suddenly have BPH or prostate cancer. The symptoms that prompt us to make the phone call to our doctor, or the problems that tests detect (on the rare occasion that we don't have symptoms first), point to a long, slow process of deterioration. For many men, the prostate gland just happens to be where that deterioration sets in. Many men have other problems as well. If we can see disease as a long, slow path away from optimal health, and if we can get to the root causes of disease, then we are well on our way to taking the steps necessary to prevent it.

Left to its devices, the body doesn't just start to go haywire for no reason. There are some common root causes for chronic diseases. We need to ask the question, "Why?" when it comes to any chronic disease, and this includes prostate disease. Research is starting to point in the direction of some of the pitfalls of our modern lifestyle: diet, stress, being sedentary, and so on. If we take a good look at what and how we eat and move and live in general, then we are well on our way to prevention.

Recall that prevention is not detection. Prevention is 1) not taking your health for granted and 2) making health priority #1 every day through

- *Healthy eating,* which includes
  - *Adding natural supplements* to counter the effects of "the modern life" (I discuss this below)
- *Exercise*
- *Managing stress* (from our busy lives and the environment)
- *Getting plenty of rest,* and
- *Doing things we enjoy,* like getting outdoors or spending time with family and friends.

Time and again I have seen this: when men make health priority #1 and shift their diet and lifestyle to improve prostate health, their overall health improves at the same time. This overall health boost gives a double boost to your prostate. Not only are you making the changes necessary to optimize your prostate health, but also when your overall health is in good order, then your immune system is stronger. A stronger immune system means your body's ability to ward off disease or mend from it is much improved. The body—if looked after with proper nutrition and lifestyle—has immense capabilities to be healthy and to repair itself and withstand disease. So how do you optimize your body's health for a healthy prostate?

FIRST, TAKE LIFE IN YOUR OWN HANDS

I often use an analogy to explain how most of us approach our body and health. Let's call it the car analogy. Most of us may not be too bothered about how our car works. We just expect it to go. If it doesn't, then we take it to the garage where a mechanic diagnoses and fixes the problem, and then we're back on the road.

Many of us treat our body the same way. We just expect it to work. That's what I mean by taking for granted our health, because most of us move through our daily lives without feeling hindered in any way by our body—until something goes wrong. Then we wheel it into the doctor; the doctor diagnoses the problem and proscribes something from his toolbox of treatments or sends us to a specialist who will use a different, more specialized set of tools. Just like the mechanic, the doctor tells you what needs to be done, and then with your permission, he or she does it.

In the case of your car, this approach should—at least in theory—be the end of your problem. But with the body, it's not so simple. Going to the doctor can be just the beginning of your problems, because, as we've seen, once a problem is detected, treatment by conventional medicine can be toxic and invasive. The side-effects can sometimes be worse to bear than the initial problem.

Now, most car mechanics will tell you what steps you can take to keep your car running smoothly, like changing the oil regularly, rotating the tires, and so on. If the mechanic can't solve the problems with your car, well, you can always sell it and buy another one. But you don't have that option with your body. So, it makes sense to pay close attention to what makes your body tick and how to keep it (and your prostate!) healthy.

Prevention begins with what we put in our mouths—the food we eat. The same analogy about cars applies to how we generally approach food. Most of us see food simply as fuel, but just as our bodies are not machines, our food is not fuel. Good nutrition is the foundation for health, and this foundation is not based on building blocks of fuel so much as it's based on a variety of nutrients. What we are aiming toward for optimal health is a "nutrient-rich" diet.

The work of prevention doesn't stop at nutrition though. We need to move our bodies through exercise. We need to manage the inevitable stress of our lives. That stress is both internal and external. Internal stress has everything to do with our fast-paced lives. External stress has to do with all the toxins and sensory overload that we are exposed to everyday. These internal and external stressors are what I mean when I say, "the effects of modern life." Natural supplements augment a health program, countering these stressors and boosting our diets by adding nutrients we don't normally find in foods available at the grocery store. For instance, many of the botanical herbs in the dietary supplements we provide at Ben's Natural Health are not commonly found in even the healthiest diet, so they literally supplement what we don't eat even when we are eating a nutrient-rich diet. For optimal health, we can (and should) address all these factors every day, as well as rest and play.

Taking these steps is our responsibility. At least as mainstream medicine is practiced today, it's not likely that your doctor is going to sit down and show you how to prevent the problem for which you sit there now hoping for a cure. Your doctor—even if he understands what needs to change about your diet and lifestyle—cannot make these changes for you or me. He cannot exercise for us. He cannot manage our stress and the environments in which we live. Doctors can do one or both of two things: 1) prescribe a pill, or more, to relieve the symptoms, and 2) operate. These measures cannot make you healthier. Only you can do that. Ultimately, your life is in your hands.

#1

DIET: THE SINGLE MOST IMPORTANT FACTOR FOR A HEALTHY PROSTATE

Very few people could be persuaded to sprinkle a little arsenic or cyanide on their bowl of cereal in the morning. Most people know that it would be something they could do only once. But every day people eat one or more things akin to sprinkling a tiny dose of poison on their food. This sprinkling adds up over time and sets into motion all kinds of problems in the body. By way of a whole cascade of "downstream" processes that we discuss in this second part of the guide, these sprinklings eventually bring about inflammation in the body, which means also, of course, in the prostate.

These "sprinklings" are the countless unhealthy foods that make up the standard diet in the West, sometimes referred to as the Standard American Diet, or SAD, or the Western Pattern Diet (WPD). The SAD is poisoning us. It is laden with sugar, processed and packaged foods loaded with chemical additives and preservatives, and meats and dairy products plagued with pharmaceuticals and excess hormones.

OUR SAD DIET

The average American gets 63% of daily calories from packaged foods. Another 25% comes from animal products, much of which is packaged, as with deli meats. That leaves only 12% of the average American daily intake for fresh vegetables, fruits, nuts and seeds, and so on. These latter foods are the fresh plant-based foods that are so nutrient rich. In addition, Americans are actually consuming more food calories than ever before. Contagious marketing campaigns by the food industry are a huge culprit for the way we eat today. How many food advertisements have you seen that sell "big" this or "mega" that? Portion sizes are larger than ever before. Have you ever noticed the difference between the size of a dinner plate today and that of 20 or even 50 years ago?

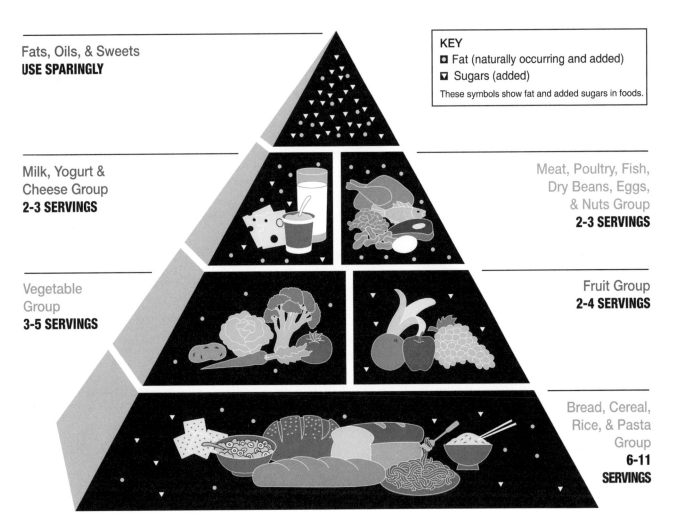

Fats, Oils, & Sweets
USE SPARINGLY

KEY
☐ Fat (naturally occurring and added)
☑ Sugars (added)
These symbols show fat and added sugars in foods.

Milk, Yogurt & Cheese Group
2-3 SERVINGS

Meat, Poultry, Fish, Dry Beans, Eggs, & Nuts Group
2-3 SERVINGS

Vegetable Group
3-5 SERVINGS

Fruit Group
2-4 SERVINGS

Bread, Cereal, Rice, & Pasta Group
6-11 SERVINGS

Source: U.S. Department of Agriculture/U.S. Department of Health and Human Services (1992 FDA Food Guide)

To make matters worse, the food industry throws a bounty of sugar-laden soft drinks, packaged desserts, and salty snack foods our way and makes them not only hard to resist, but addictive even! Marion Nestle, Ph.D., professor of Nutrition, Food Studies, and Public Health at New York University, writes in her book, Food Politics: How the Food Industry Influences Nutrition and Health, "It can hardly be a coincidence that these are just the foods that are most profitable to the food industry and that it most vigorously promotes." No wonder we are seeing surging rates of obesity and a growing epidemic of chronic diseases!

Let's talk about processed foods for a moment since this "food group" makes up the overwhelming majority of the average diet in the US and UK. Walk down most of the aisles of your supermarket and you will see that with the exception of fresh produce, the rest of the food is packaged. Some exceptions can be found in grocery stores that have a "bulk" section where you have the option to choose from a variety of nuts, seeds, and grains to dispense into bags in whatever quantity you choose. Even in the bulk section, though, you will find an ever-increasing number of prepared or processed foods, such as "sesame sticks," rice crackers, and even vegetable chips. And if your supermarket has a butcher or fishmonger section, you will see animal foods that are not packaged. The remainder of what you see in the grocery store comes packaged and more often than not prepared and processed.

Prepared foods and processed foods are not necessarily the same. When we buy fresh vegetables at the market, we may go through any number of steps to prepare them for a meal: wash, peel, slice or chop, cook, and so on. We may buy freshly prepared foods from a restaurant or market deli. Bear in mind that not all prepared foods are created equally. Processed food, on the other hands, has gone through a whole host of … processes … to turn it into a product that often barely resembles the original food source. Cheese-flavored chips or crackers, for instance, are a far cry, when it comes to ingredients, from the description of them.

Let's zoom in for a minute and take a closer look at processed foods. You likely don't have to walk down the aisles of your local supermarket to find an example or two. Most of us will find plenty of processed foods in our own pantries and fridges. These foods are appealing because they are convenient.

#1

First, the flours that go into store-bought breads, cereals, crackers, cookies, and so on—staples of most households—are grains that have been finely ground into powder and fortified with added vitamins and minerals. The manufacturing process took out some of the healthiest parts of the grains where the vitamins and minerals are found. Turning grains into flour reduces them to simple starches. Starches are so quickly metabolized by the body and turned into glucose (the form of sugar that the body uses) that they cause a sudden spike in insulin (the hormone that clears sugar from the blood to store it for later use as energy), which, over the long haul, can create insulin resistance.

#2

Second, and on top of the starch issue, the majority of these foods have added sweeteners, particularly cookies and cereals—not just sugar, but honey, maple syrup, and worse, processed sweeteners like high fructose corn syrup, dextrose, and so on. When we take in too much sugar and starches for the body to use immediately, insulin production skyrockets to transfer the glucose into the liver and muscles where it will be stored until needed.

#3

Processed sweeteners, such as high fructose corn syrup, along with juice sweeteners are not taken up by the body in the same way as starches and sugar. They bypass the insulin spike, being metabolized instead by the liver. When the body does not have an immediate need for these sugars, the liver stores them as fat. They also have the added effect of bypassing the body's natural appetite suppressor, which says, "I've had enough. I think I'll stop eating cookies now." Without this natural "stop" signal, we are inclined to keep eating these foods.

What's more, the majority of processed foods contain additives that are flavor enhancers. With just the right amount of flavor enhancer, a packaged food becomes almost irresistible once we start eating or drinking it! Our "stop" signal has been overpowered, and if we do manage to put down the package for this sitting, we are sure to go back to it, creating a cycle of unhealthy eating.

STANDARD American DIET

The problem is that with the SAD and an increasingly sedentary lifestyle, we don't need this surplus of sugar. Over time, the cells' receptors to insulin become less sensitive to it, excess energy is stored as fat, and the liver gets sluggish. When insulin resistance happens, the cells cannot take up the excess sugar. Now, the pancreas produces more insulin to assist with moving the sugar into storage. The more resistant the cells become to insulin, the more sugar that is "free-floating" in the bloodstream. This excess contributes to inflammation in the body, which can become chronic and give way to the development of diseases, including diabetes and ... yes, prostate disease. What's more, cancer cells thrive on sugar!

Third, these processed foods contain a glut of stabilizers and preservatives that extend the shelf-life of these products and also make them more appealing—mostly through food coloring. Some of these additives are "excitotoxins" that make the product appeal to our taste buds just so that we will continue eating them. Monosodium glutamate (MSG) is one such food additive that enhances flavor and ropes us in to addiction to that particular food.

These chemical additives are not food-based, and many of them are anti-microbial, which means they not only limit the growth of bacteria and other microbes in the packaged food to keep them from rotting, but they also do a number on the microbes that keep our guts healthy. The end result is a chemical concoction that has little or no nutritional value, but it makes you think and feel that you have eaten. Worst of all, it provides the lowest grade materials for your body and adds toxins that your body struggles to get rid of. The point I want to make here is that, like starches and sugar, which fall into the category of "carbs" (carbohydrates), these chemical additives also cause inflammation in the body, which means inflammation in the prostate. *CaRBS: STARCHES & Sugar*

I've purposefully oversimplified all the processes that take place in the body when we consume starches, sugars, and food additives to make a point, which is this: the SAD is poisoning us. It puts us at significant risk for developing chronic disease, but, as I have emphasized, chronic diseases are not inevitable. Shifting away from the SAD will dramatically reduce your risk of developing prostate disease.

YOU ARE WHAT YOUR FOOD EATS: SOME HAZARDS OF MODERN EATING

SAD= Standard American Diet

Let's talk now about the second most prevalent group of foods in the SAD diet: animal products. These include fresh and packaged meats, milk and cheese, butter, and eggs, as well as seafood. Unfortunately, the majority of these animal products come from sickly animals raised in intensely confined areas of industrialized "farms"—called CAFOs (concentrated animal feeding operation). CAFOs produce the bulk of the meat consumed in the US. These operations "turn out" a large number of animals quickly on very small parcels of land, making this industrial form of agriculture an intense method of animal production for an ever-expanding global population that is also increasingly meat-focused.

There are significant problems with these animal operations. CAFO animals are pumped full of hormones to make them grow faster or make more milk. They are also loaded with antibiotics to ward off disease because their living conditions are so crowded and horrific that they would die otherwise. This is not an exaggerated point. Most of these animals have no room to turn around and stand or sit in excrement all day and night. As if the hormones and antibiotics in the meats and dairy products are not problematic enough, these animals are constantly stressed in such living conditions, and the stress hormones (cortisol) coursing through their bodies make their way into the meat and milk we consume. When we eat those animal products, we are also eating their stress hormones, which are then absorbed into our bloodstream.

And just as concerning, CAFO animals are eating foods that their bodies can't process. For instance, CAFOs feed grain-corn to cows to fatten them up—fast. Without grain, cow meat does not develop the marbled quality that many people have come expect as "good" red meat. But cows are grass-eating animals. Corn does such a number on their guts that all the CAFO cows around the globe produce more CO_2 from flatulence than all the automobiles on the highway! When cows graze on grass, however, their meat and milk contain "micro-nutrients" that cannot be found in corn-fed cows, and these grass-grazing cows' meat also contains a higher percentage of omega-3 fatty acids.

Similarly, caged chickens fed a diet of only grains produce eggs that are less nutritious than chickens scratching at the ground, eating what these "yard birds" like to eat and natural to them: a wide variety of grasses and clovers, insects, worms, and so on. Like pastured cows, pastured chickens produce eggs that are higher in omega-3 fatty acids, a key component of the modified KETO diet, which I discuss later. Pastured eggs are also higher in vitamin E, a natural antioxidant that helps to counter inflammation.

omega-3 Fatty acids
Vit E

Lastly on the animal list: fish and seafood. The most pressing concern about eating fish, either farm-raised or wild-caught, is the quality of water in which these animals live and eat. Oceans have become a dumping ground of industrial waste and human consumerism. Heavy metals can be a concern when eating a diet high in seafood. In general, the larger the fish, the more likely it is to have higher concentrations of heavy metals, such as mercury, for instance. Farm-raised fish are also subject to the quality of water in which they live. Because these fish-farms are "closer to home," the water can be more tainted than deep, open ocean waters, particularly those closer to the arctic or Antarctica.

The point I want to emphasize here is that what animals eat, we eat. Not only is over-prescribing antibiotics in a medical setting a public health risk, making it harder for us to fight infections, but so too is consuming a diet high in meats from CAFOs. To make matters worse, the antibiotics in animal meats wreak havoc on the healthy bacteria in our guts—our microbiome. The microbiome has taken center stage in research over the past decade for its importance in helping with digesting food, warding off infection, and producing vital vitamins and chemical transmitters that support our mood, lessen our response to stress, boost our immune system, and help maintain our overall health. Any insult to the microbiome sets into motion a long and winding river of downstream effects on our health.

Before you put this guide down, depressed and despairing about the state of affairs I have just presented about the foods you likely love, I encourage you to read on. Very shortly our attention will turn to the safe and healthy, easy, affordable, satisfying, and delicious changes you can make to your diet starting today that take into consideration these concerns. For now, though, hang in there, and let's consider together what that third group of foods on the SAD diet eats: plants. What do they "eat"?

Plants take their nutrients from sun, water, earth, and air. As far as I know, the sun is not likely to come under the influence of modern human life anytime soon! Water, earth, and air do, however. Conventional farming relies on fertilizers and pesticides to produce bountiful crops. As with industrial animal farming techniques, these conventional plant farming methods can pose risks to our health.

Fertilizers add to the soil what is not there but essential for the plant to thrive. These fertilizers add one to three, or a grouping of minerals, typically nitrogen, phosphorus, and potassium. Plants cannot grow without these three "macro-nutrients." Some plants require other elements. Beets, for instance, require boron in the soil for the plant to produce a fat beetroot. We humans, on the other hand, require many more minerals than plants in order to be healthy. We need a host of "micro-nutrients," such as zinc, magnesium, selenium, and boron that occur in smaller amounts or not at all in conventionally grown produce.

Pesticides are used by farmers to keep weeds at bay, as well as insects feeding on the plants, and fungi, especially during particularly wet growing seasons. Pesticides kill anything that may negatively affect the cultivated plants but not the plants themselves. And some farmers use pesticides to kill the actual cultivated plants just before harvest to make crop-picking more efficient. Potato farmers use this pre-harvest technique. When pesticides are sprayed on plants and their fruits, residues remain, which are not easily washed away under the tap. Eating plants sprayed with pesticides brings with it a host of potential health risks. Some pesticides have been linked to cancer. Also, the impact on our healthy gut bacteria is immediate and significant. These chemicals kill the healthy bacteria in our guts. In recent years, of course, scientists have come up with genetic manipulation to further change our food and allow for more intensive farming.

Not one of these changes has been done in order to improve the nutritional value of the foods. Companies are making huge sums of money with these modified crops and organisms. We should be very wary of eating them, because so far, there is enough evidence to suggest, in my opinion, that these genetic modifications are linked to potential health problems.

WHY YOU ARE WHAT YOU EAT

Our body is made up of trillions of cells! These cells are constantly changing. Each day millions of cells die and are replaced with new ones. Each second of life there are billions of biochemical processes and interactions taking place inside and between the cells to keep you alive, enable you to grow, think, function, walk, talk, digest food, have sex, produce babies, repel infection, and repair damage. In fact, cellular renewal is so extensive that over every seven-year period, virtually all the cells in the body are completely replaced. This means that every seven years you become a totally new person!

So where does our body source the energy to sustain and continually recreate itself? Well, partly by the air we breathe. But the greatest make-up of our body is the food we eat and of course, the water that we drink.

If we imagine for just a moment that the body is like a self-manufacturing house, we can see that each bit of food is like material for the structure the body is self-building. It will cope when receiving materials that are not ideally suited to its structure by using them instead of the materials that it would ideally call on. Each substitution with low-grade materials, however, will reduce the resiliency and efficiency of the "body-house" and make it function sub-optimally. When the substitution with "low-grade materials" is too extensive or frequent, then the structure is so weakened that it begins to fail. When this happens in the body, disease follows.

What you eat therefore becomes the cellular structure and processes that make up your body. So, while you are what you eat, you are also what you do not eat. If you fill yourself with junk food, that food is taking the place of nutritious healthy food that would support a healthy cellular structure and processes. Every time we eat, we are providing materials for the self-building and self-maintaining "body-house." Junk materials may not make for a sturdy house, and they certainly won't weather a storm. The body is extraordinarily adaptable, but it is also only as healthy as what we put into it.

Fascinatingly, despite the fact that the US is the wealthiest country in the world, increasing numbers of people are malnourished, so much so that large numbers of people in the US are more malnourished than populations in developing countries! For many people, this malnourishment problem in the US is not a question of what they can afford. It is a question of what so many people choose to eat. This is not the case for everyone, of course. Unfortunately, the cheapest food on the market is processed food with all the addictive qualities of a pack of cigarettes. The food industry spends countless dollars on marketing unhealthy foods. What you eat can look like food, smell like food, even taste like food, but, as I have emphasized above, so often there is very little real food in many of the choices we have before us at the supermarket,

"You are what you eat" is a stronger incentive than ever before for going back to basics. Buy only real food. Stay away from processed, canned, wrapped, frozen, or packaged food products. Look at the ingredients on the packaging label if you must buy a packaged product. If you see any item on the list that you do not recognize as food, then put the package away.

I talk more later about choosing organic over conventional, grass-fed and pasture-raised animals over industrialized animal products, and so on. But even switching away from processed food to fresh foods is a huge step in the direction of improving your health. Learn how to prepare fresh foods and take your health back into your own hands.

A HUNDRED YEARS OF CHANGES IN WESTERN DIET & LIFESTYLE

How, you might ask, *did we get here? Haven't people always eaten this way, save for the processed and junk foods?* Well, yes and no. There is no doubt that many of the staples of the Western diet have a long history as mainstays. Certainly, we would find plenty of evidence of and recipes from centuries ago illustrating the place of breads and grain cereals, roasted meats, and sweets in our ancestors' diets. But a lot has changed over the past century to drastically alter our food, as well as our habits and traditions. A hundred years ago, the global population was 1.8 billion people. In 2018, it is 7.6 billion people and projected to reach over 9 billion by 2030. This steep, upward trend of population growth is like nothing the world has ever seen before. As a result, our methods of growing and producing food turned to more production-intensive methods. What we gain in quantity, however, we sacrifice in the quality. And this is so for several reasons.

WWII's Effects on Today's Western Diet

During World War II, with multiple coordinated efforts to feed the large numbers of troops on the battlefront, not only were families at home required to ration dietary staples like sugar, butter, meat, and coffee. Factories in the US and Europe also responded to a call from the military to develop foods for troops. These processed and packaged products were to be high in fat and calories (energy!) and able to withstand the harsh conditions that troops on the front lines endured. The food industry heeded the call, introducing new energy-packed foods to add to troops' food ration packs.

Energy-Packed Processed Foods

It is not that preserving and packaging food was new to the WWII era. It is that WWII and the years that followed tipped off an explosion of processed food and a new interest in convenience. The extent to which the needs of the military and food corporations eager to make a profit conspired to create lightweight, calorie-dense foods cannot be overstated. Military research in the transport of blood plasma, for instance, set the course for the development of instant coffee to also make its way to the battlefields. The military's interest in "fabricated modules of meat" eventually paved the way for McDonald's brand McRib®, and the orange residue on Cheetos® has its beginnings in 1943 when a dehydrated and compressed "cheese" was invented to send to troops.

A Market for Convenience

After the war, the wheels of food-processing were already turning. A host of new products became popular like Spam® and M&Ms®, for instance. With so many men at war, women had entered the workforce headlong. Now they wanted to keep their jobs! And food processors found a new market: the general public. Packaged foods began to fill a convenience need for working women who had husbands and children to feed at the end of a long workday. And so began the surging market for tasty, packaged, and increasingly convenient foods.

New foods brought about novel flavors and taste preferences. Rather than home-baked, whole-grain breads, now consumers preferred packaged and sliced "white" bread. Early preservation methods had relied largely on salt and sugar. But now manufacturers wanted to advance the plot: reduce the amount of water in foods as much as possible so they would be less likely to spoil. This effort brought about lab-based chemical additives. Food colorings were added for visual appeal. Each stage of the food packaging and processing development ushered in foods increasingly removed from their original source, and with this arc of change, evermore unhealthy adulterations.

A Green Revolution

The post-WWII era also ushered in a "Green Revolution." Munitions factories with excess nitrogen used in explosives were suddenly without a war-time need to produce explosives. With a good dose of research and development, many of these factories turned to manufacturing fertilizers from the nitrogen ammonium and other petroleum-based products found in ammunition. They turned their marketing attention to local farmers who had already oriented themselves toward intensive production during the wartime food shortages. Farmers began using these agro-chemicals. Very shortly, they saw bounty from their fields like never before.

But with more intense farming, the soil became depleted. Crops became more susceptible to disease and "pests." The old munitions factories answered this new pest problem with an entire armament of pesticides: insecticides for bugs, herbicides for weeds that might choke out good crops, and fungicides for "blight." With the Cold War stirring fears of another world war, along with explosive population growth worldwide, agriculture pushed for higher yielding crops and farming technologies that could be exported to developing countries.

Excess Grain

This new brigade of agricultural technologies brought about a surplus of food, the likes of which the West had never seen. That surplus was largely in the form of grains. By the late 50s and early 60s, the US was floating in a sea of excess, mostly corn, wheat, rye, and oats.

With high-yielding grains to spare and sugar cane tariffs in place, scientists developed a technique to convert the starch from corn into fructose, which is the sugar found in fruits. Soon, high fructose corn syrup (HFCS) started to replace beet and cane sugar in most packaged products, and between 1975 and 2000, there was a 25% increase in "added sugars" in packaged foods. Not surprisingly, obesity rates surged, as did diabetes.

The Food Pyramid & Grain across the Food Chain

Whether or not the wealth of grain in the US contributed to the development of the Food Pyramid in the late 80s is debatable. But it is interesting to note that the two coincide. While the food pyramid, with its recommendation of 6–11 servings per day of grains, including breads, cereals, pasta, will feed a growing population worldwide, it is also a dietary guideline that works in favor of farmers and food manufacturers—farmers who have surplus grains and food manufacturers who have cheap access to them and aim to turn a profit. And although the Food Pyramid has been replaced recently by the "My Plate" guidelines in the US, most middle-aged Americans were "raised on" the Food Pyramid guidelines. The majority of us still think it is the healthiest way to eat. But there is a growing body of research now that tells us this is not so.

U.S GOVERNMENT "MY PLATE" DIETARY RECCOMMENDATION

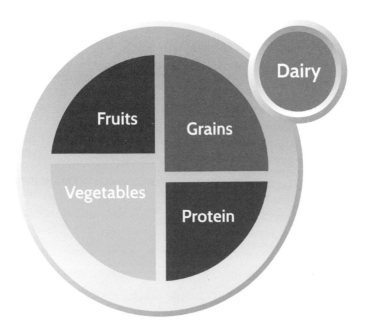

Also, most of the fresh meats and packaged animal products found today in the standard supermarket come from animals fed and fattened up on these excess grains, as I explained above. Grains cheapen not only the cost of mass animal agriculture, but they also cheapen the quality of meat. Just like us, these animals need a variety of green, grassy plants. When they eat mostly grains, their milk and meat are not as vitamin and mineral rich as it is when they eat a variety of grasses. In fact, some vital nutrients, such as Vitamin K2 can only be found in the milk and meat of pastured grass-eating animals.

We need to pay closer attention to the nutrition science than to dietary guidelines, which can be tainted by the complicated politics of food and the interests of giant food corporations.

Changing Habits & Traditions

Not only have the food industry and the changing tides of the past 100 years influenced what we eat, but our habits and traditions have also changed how we eat. Our desire for convenience and access to cheapened ingredients and fast foods wrecks what we eat, and our ever-increasing pace of work and life keeps us from enjoying the pleasure of preparing healthy meals and eating them with friends and loved ones. So many people in the US and UK barely know how to prepare a fresh meal today, relying instead on restaurant or ready-to-eat packaged meals. In short, for most of us, our what and how of eating is at the heart of the chronic diseases epidemic—70% of all diseases now are considered to be chronic and related to our modern lifestyle. Prostate disease, as I have indicated, is among them.

Our Hurried Lives

With the demands of longer work-days, lengthy commutes, and the majority of households relying on income from all adults living at home, as well as time-commitments outside of home and work, our lives are, in a word, rushed. Gone are the days of mostly home-cooked meals. The majority of people in the US and Europe now eat about half of their meals out, which also includes calling on delivery services. For those who do eat at home, ready-to-eat packaged meals take second place to restaurant foods.

In fact, the majority of people living in the US spend more than 40% of their food dollars on eating out, and depending on age and income brackets, most of these food dollars are from fast or quick-service food. A 2012–2013 USDA survey revealed that most respondents who relied on fast food were younger and employed with children, and they also tended to have a higher body mass index (overweight or obese). Those from the same survey who did not rely on eating out and ready-made meals tended to be older and living in more rural settings where convenience foods were not as accessible.

The problem with this habit is that restaurant foods, particularly fast-food restaurants, and pre-packaged meals, as we have seen, are not prepared with nutrition in mind. They are appealing because they are convenient, quick, and tasty, and they allow us to get back to our hurried lives. There is very little about this growing trend away from freshly prepared meals that actually feeds us well and supports our health.

Eating at Work

Over 30 million Americans skip breakfast every day, according to a recent NPD survey. The reasons most people say they do so are either that they are not hungry yet (before going to work) or that they are too busy and rushed. Then, when lunchtime comes around, the majority of us eat at our desks, in front of a computer, browsing social media or something similar for half an hour before getting back to work—or worse, working straight through lunch. The same is true for dinner. Increasingly, people eat in front of a screen. And we are more likely to eat alone than we are to eat with others. These eating habits also pull us into the convenience of packaged, processed food.

Unless we have developed a practice of intermittent fasting, which I discuss later, skipping breakfast puts us at risk for grabbing something mid-morning to stave off hunger until lunch. This mid-morning snack, more often than not, ends up being a spur-of-the-moment purchase from an office vending-machine or a nearby coffee shop. Either way, prioritizing good nutrition is thrown out the window for the effort to quiet the belly. When we are hungry enough and haven't planned for it, even our best nutrition intentions are cast aside.

In a different and slower time, lunch was the main meal of the day. People almost always ate this mid-day meal with family. Conversation slowed eating enough to allow the body to register "I'm full." Many Europeans still break for mid-day meals. Shops close. Families go home for lunch and enjoy a mid-day break for up to two hours. They also tend to work into the evening to off-set the mid-day break, whereas in the US, the pace just keeps getting more hurried and the work-day more packed. Scientists speculate that this difference in work and eating habits may be a reason many European countries have lower rates of obesity than that of the United States.

Of course, with the hustle and buzz of our work-a-day life in the US, this mid-day lunch break is easier said than done. Eating the largest meal of the day at lunch is a far cry from the American norm. Most of us have experienced that doing so puts us at risk for being tired in the afternoon. While our US work day is probably not going to change any time soon, on a personal level, and with a little work and support from friends and family who may wish to try out a new way of living along with you, it is possible to change your eating habits. You might try at least stepping away from the computer screen, relaxing a bit, and slowing down, if for only that 30-minute lunch break.

Eating a lighter meal at dinner gives your body a leg up on digestion before you go to bed, which is when many people struggle with indigestion. Heavy meals mean slower digestion. When eaten at dinner, your body is still breaking down the food in your belly when you crawl into bed. This is when people experience "heartburn." Lying down with a belly full of fatty food is bound to put backward pressure on the contents of the stomach. It is better to eat these heavier meals earlier in the day when the body will have plenty of time to digest them.

Eating while Staring at a Screen

Staring at a computer, TV, or telephone screen pulls our attention away from our meal and important cues from our bodies. Have you ever noticed after eating a meal when you were so distracted by what you were watching that you missed tasting your food? We tend to become so engrossed in what is taking place on our screens that we scarcely notice that we are eating! We shovel it in, and often hurriedly. Eating too quickly bypasses the body's natural "Stop. I'm full" warning system.

It takes, on average, about twenty minutes for your brain to recognize that you are full. Receptors in the stomach and brain signal us to stop eating. But if we are eating so quickly that we have shoveled in more than the natural appetite threshold before the body can register it, then we have just overeaten. Too much of this way of eating, and we find the pounds adding up. That's why you can eat much more if you eat quickly.

We do not have teeth inside our guts, so slowing down, and chewing, is an essential part of healthy eating. I know. You've heard this before—since you were a little kid. This time, Mom was right. Chewing incorporates important enzymes from saliva that together begin the food-breakdown process. Failure to chew thoroughly reduces the effectiveness of the digestive process and is likely to lead to indigestion.

Let's look at an example. A dinner-plate sized pancake with butter is a full meal for most people. After eating one of those, the average person is probably not likely to have a second one. If you stack two or even three of these pancakes on top of each other and eat them all together, you'll probably not only get them all down in one sitting, but also, you probably won't notice that you are full until after you've finished. Had you had just one pancake on your plate and eaten it slowly, you likely would have recognized that you were full long before reaching for that second or third pancake.

In fact, we only fully taste the first mouthful. Each mouthful that follows lacks the quality of exciting the palate in the same way that the first mouthful did. This means that the amount you eat does not enhance the pleasure element. Yes, each next bite does not taste better than that first one. So, relish that first mouthful to the maximum, and do not believe that eating more will be more enjoyable. Each bite is a chase for the pleasure we experienced at the first bite. The first mouthful is for enjoyment, the other mouthfuls for nutrition, and more is not necessarily better.

Eating More . . . and Eating More Sweets

About 65% of Americans are overweight, and 35% are obese, whereas in the 1970s, about 14% of Americans were considered to be obese. These numbers go hand-in-hand with an increase in the amount of food consumed that I discussed above. Americans now eat on average about 425 more calories per day than 50 years ago. This number reflects an increase across most types of food, but it is particularly true for sugary beverages.

Food manufacturers developed soft drinks more than a century ago. Today, these drinks contain much more sugar than those earlier versions and provide a substantial amount of sugar in the American diet. The average American now drinks the equivalent of one 16-ounce soft drink every day, to the tune of about 43 grams or nearly 3 tablespoons of sugar! This glut amounts to about 1/10th of a pound with each 16-ounce soda. If you were to drink just one of these drinks every day of the year, you would consume more than 35 pounds of sugar each year in soft drinks alone.

Let's put these numbers into some perspective. In the mid-1700s the average American consumed about 4 pounds of sugar each year. A hundred years later in the mid-1800s, that American would have consumed about 20 pounds of sugar each year. A hundred and fifty years later, at the turn of the 21st century, this same "average" American consumed more than 160 pounds of sugar each year! Clearly, sugary soft drinks are a big part of this sugar number, but they are not the whole story. Added sugar can be found in almost every type of packaged food. It shows up in the strangest of places. If you look at the food labels in your pantry or fridge, you will see added sugars in the forms of concentrated fruit juice, corn syrup, high fructose corn syrup, sugar, honey, maple syrup, sucrose, dextrose, and fructose.
The graph below shows that the average American consumes between 100 and 120 pounds of sugar each year.

Eating More Red Meat

According to National Health and Nutrition Examination Surveys (NHANES), the average American eats about 100 pounds of meat per year, excluding fish. That's twice as much meat as people ate a century ago. While trends are similar in the UK and Europe, the US is the largest consumer of meat worldwide, and red meat is the largest source of meat consumed.

U.S. Sugar Consumption
1907-2017

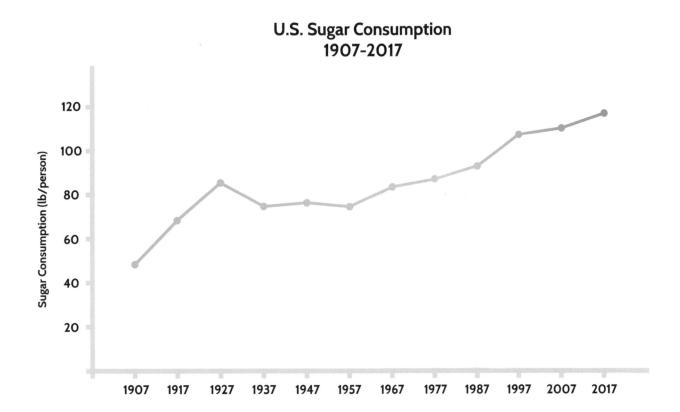

Total U.S. Meat Consumption

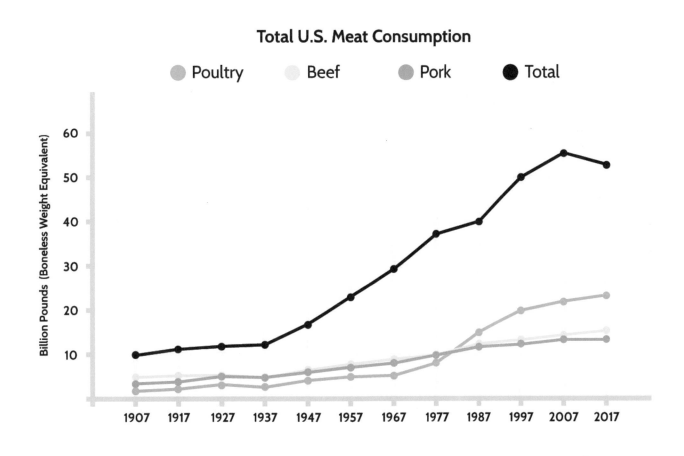

Meat provides protein, important fat-soluble vitamins and minerals, and fats. But consuming a high-meat diet can be problematic too. First, the overwhelming majority of meat consumed in the US and UK is processed meat. Meat processors cure meat with salts and chemicals, such as nitrates and nitrites, which have been linked to colon cancer. Smoking and grilling meat can also produce cancer-causing compounds. So many of the ways that we are accustomed to enjoying meat can pose health risks. Braising, poaching, and baking fresh cuts of meat reduce these risks, as does avoiding smoked, cured, and processed, packaged meats (luncheon meats) altogether.

You will recall from above that there are hosts of problems with the way that animals are being raised now. Cheap grain-corn in animal feed has made for cheaper meat, percentage wise, to what it was even 50 years ago. Fast-food restaurants have capitalized on this cheaper meat and encouraged our appetites for it. And it's not only Americans and Europeans who are hungry to enjoy the pleasures of animal fare.

see page 59

When we eat animals that are raised in CAFOs, we are eating all the antibiotics and hormones that have been fed to them, which challenge our body's immune system and natural hormone balance. And, as I said before, grain-fed meats have a different composition of fatty acids than pastured animals, which have higher amounts of healthy omega-3 fatty acids. Also, many of these meats are processed with antimicrobial chemicals during the washing and packing stages, which, again, make their way into our bodies. The point is that industrialized meat practices, as well as processed and fast-food meats, are an obstacle to good health. We should avoid them if at all possible.

On the other hand, animals raised on farms that use "animal-centered," humane practices and allow their animals to graze and freely roam pastures provide meats that fortify our health. Rich in healthy nutrients not found in CAFO animals, these meats are also lacking in all the chemicals and pharmaceuticals that contaminate "conventional" agriculture meats. If you have access to a good farmer's market, or better yet, if you know farmers who raise animals in pastures where they are free to roam and graze, buy from them. You will be astonished at the difference in these meats—their color, texture, and flavor, and when properly prepared, they will become a boost to your healthy diet.

A word of caution: be careful about the label "grass-fed" that has become a new marketing ploy. Industrial agriculture knows what sells. They are just as quick to put grass in the animal feed at their CAFOs and call their meat "grass-fed" as they are to tout the flavor of "corn-fed" meats because corn is cheap, after all. It is best to know your farmer, and if that is not possible, find a good butcher who insists on sourcing meat from farmers who use "humane" practices. Whether you are concerned about how the animals are raised is not the point I am making about farming practices. The point I am making is that healthy animals equal healthy meats.

Drinking More Alcohol

Alcohol consumption has gone through trends, sometimes rising and sometimes falling. That said, there has definitely been an uptick in the US over the past decade. Theories abound about why, including the global recession that plagued not only the US economy, but that of the entire globe. So many people still have not recovered. And these are frighteningly uncertain times. People tend to turn to alcohol and other substances to cope.

Alcohol is a toxin. Although we may enjoy it casually and socially, our body receives it as something akin to a poison. The words "toxin" and "intoxicant" are similar for a reason. As soon as the alcohol passes through the walls of the intestine, the body begins filtering it through the liver.

While some studies show that moderate consumption of red wine or other drinks can have protective effects on blood vessels and can slow or prevent the development of cardiovascular disease, it is important to understand that alcohol provides no real nutritional value. Because it is broken down and processed in the liver, drinking alcohol can lead to the development of a fatty liver or cirrhosis. In addition, many cocktails, as well as wine, contain large amounts of sugar. The combined alcohol and sugar stimulate inflammation and the problems that come with that—including, as is hopefully obvious by now . . . prostate disease.

Lastly, it is much easier to engage in unhealthy eating habits with or after a few drinks. Whatever discipline we may have mustered to focus on our health flies out the window. To make matters worse, for many people, these eating–drinking "slips" take place at night. So, on top of going to bed shortly after eating, a problem we've already discussed, your body now has the added task of breaking down and filtering out the alcohol. This process also contributes to weight gain from drinking, typically around the waist.

U.S Average of Alcohol Consumption

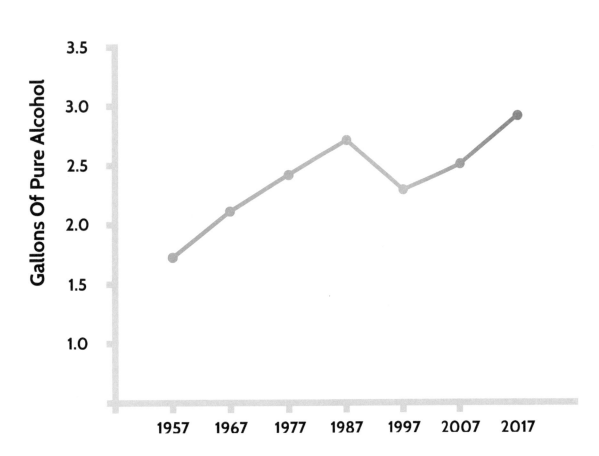

Eating Late & Sleep

Our biological clocks have also changed. We live in a world that never stops. Billions of people work all hours of the day or night to keep the global economy and our local emergency, law enforcement, and healthcare systems going. Those of us working nights or worse, changing shifts from day to night and back again, are constantly challenged to find a stable sleep–wake rhythm, which puts the body into a perpetual state of stress. Many others of us have steady hours but, with the increasing demands of work, get off later and later, working routinely into the evening—after sitting all day.

Our work/life balance is so out of whack that we can hardly manage to find the time or energy to take care of our health. It is making our health a priority—over work, even—that we need to change radically. I'm not saying that we need to quit our jobs. What I am saying is that if our work/life balance is so out of sync with caring for our health, then we need to seriously reflect on how to redesign our lives. I want to highlight again that our health is in our own hands—not in the hands of our boss or our business, or the food industry, or industrial agriculture. We need to constantly step back and look at our lives and how we spend our time and dollars.

With that, let's talk about what our bodies need when it comes to healthy sleep. Our bodies—from way, way back—expect that we will sleep when it's dark and wake up with the sun. When we get off schedule in our sleep, either by swinging shifts, traveling from one time zone to another one very different from our "home" zone, or get by on fewer than 6 hours of sleep, our bodies go into the stress response. Our bodies have not caught up to modern times completely. Any time there is a "stressor," the body responds internally in much the same way as it would have ages ago when we were living in the elements. A sudden chase by a tiger! A long, cold winter with little to no food. These old "triggers" for seeking energy are registered by the body no differently than a markedly shortened night's sleep or waking in a new time zone when we are "supposed" to be sleeping. These sleep changes stimulate the release of a cascade of hormones that increase our appetite because the body thinks it needs more energy to deal with this stressor.

Eating just before bed doesn't help matters. Our bodies want to be sleeping at night, not digesting food, which can disrupt our sleep, even if we do get to bed on time. Without a healthy sleep pattern, we are at risk of eating too much, gaining weight, and developing other stress-related problems that weaken our immune system and contribute to chronic inflammation. Later, I'll talk about ways to shift eating and sleep for better health. For now, to better your sleep and your health, you might think about simply shifting your largest meal of the day to your mid-day meal and putting away all electronic devices by dinner time.

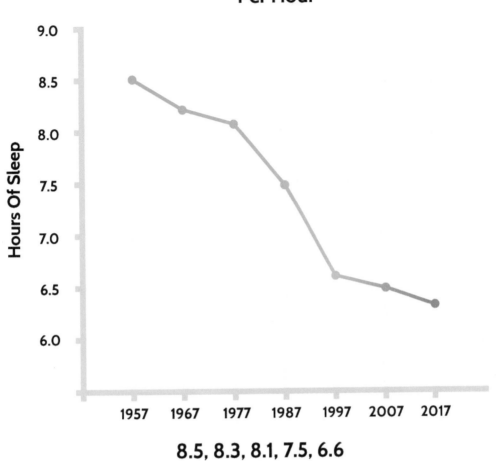

U.S. Average Amount Of Sleep Per Hour

8.5, 8.3, 8.1, 7.5, 6.6

Rolling Back the Hands of Time: The Paleolithic Diet

The past century has no doubt impacted our habits and the types of food we eat. There is plenty of evidence to show that these changes have contributed to the chronic diseases that 70% of the US population experiences today, including prostate disease. Reversing or trying to prevent prostate disease is reason enough to look at how our bodies are naturally inclined to eat.

Over the past decade, the "paleolithic diet," or "paleo diet," has captured the attention of many who want to do just this—roll back the hands of time and return to something close to hunter–gatherer ways of eating. Many people believe this way of eating might be the healthiest. The idea is that our bodies inherited characteristics that took millions of years to evolve. Most of these characteristics were handed down from the way life was before humans first began to farm.

In general, hunter–gatherers foraged for wild edible plants, fruits, seeds, nuts, and honey, and hunted wild animals. Infants and young children nursed and drank the milk of their own species, but once weaned, they no longer drank milk. When humans began keeping animals and farming about 10,000 years ago, many of the plants they successfully cultivated were cereal grains, such as corn and wheat. The "diseases of civilization" (heart disease, diabetes, thyroid and prostate disease, many cancers, and others) are thought to be the result of adding grain, dairy, and fattier meats to our diet while at the same time losing many important nutrients found in the plentiful variety of plant foods that our ancient ancestors ate.

It's important to point out here that the paleo diet is not a weight-loss plan like so many diet trends tend to be. Even so, switching from the SAD to "paleo" often leads to weight-loss because junk foods, grains, and a huge percentage of the sugar that we consume are eliminated from the paleo diet. As a result of cutting out these types of foods, paleo diet advocates say this way of eating boosts health and can reverse disease. The notion that our biology has not yet caught up with the changing pace of culture makes sense, and some researchers believe this incompatibility is at the heart of so many of today's diseases.

From farming and animal husbandry to the later use of stone-age tools for milling grains and seeds, and more recently, machines to do much of this work, every technological advancement brought about changes to our quality of food. When grains were milled using stones, for instance, all the contents of the grain were preserved, including the fiber-rich germ and bran. With the Industrial Revolution and the invention of a mechanized steel roller and machine sifters, the germ and bran were left out of the milled grain, leaving only the starchy part. This development dramatically changed the quality of the grain consumed since the Industrial Revolution. Now, of course, highly refined flours line our supermarket aisles, along with every imaginable breakfast cereal, cookie, cracker, and so on, the #1 ingredient of which is refined flour. The ingredients that follow flour on the label are typically some type of refined sugar, refined vegetable oil, and salt—none of which would have been a part of the diet of our earliest human ancestors.

Also, once humans started domesticating animals, it became possible to reduce the decrease in body fat that was inevitable in wild animals during less abundant seasons. Now they could feed animals year-round with stored grains. With farming, it was also possible to time the slaughter when body fat was at its peak. Other early technology advances allowed humans to cure and store meat, as well as render energy-rich animal fats in the forms of butter, cheese, and tallow. Fast forward to modern times and CAFO animals, which are technically obese at the time of slaughter. The same is not true for pastured animals.

Dairy products, cereal grains, refined sugars and vegetable oils, along with alcohol now make up over 70% of the total calories consumed each day by people in the US. These foods would have been absent from the diet of preagricultural humans. What does this evolution in eating mean for us today and how might these changes contribute to prostate disease?

1. A high-sugar diet, and specifically refined sugars, is perhaps the #1 cause of chronic inflammation, and disease. You will recall that chronic inflammation contributes to all forms of prostate disease: BPH, prostatitis, and prostate cancer.
2. The grain-based staples in our diet not only cause blood sugar to rise, leading to chronic inflammation and insulin resistance. Grains also effectively push out the nutrient-dense plant

foods that support healthy cell function and our immune system.

3. The reduced variety of foods that we eat today decreases nutrient intake. Although most of us would not say we are starving, many people eating the SAD are actually malnourished. Healthy bodies begin with good nutrition.

4. Dairy products also cause blood sugar and insulin levels to rise, much like starches and sugars do, and many people also suffer an immune response to the proteins in dairy, casein and whey, which adds to the inflammation that occurs with sugar intake. Dairy can also contribute to hormone imbalances, particularly estrogen. We now know that elevated levels of estrogen contribute to prostate disease.

5. Refined oils also contribute to inflammation.

6. Grain-fattened and cured animal meats don't have the rich omega-3 fatty acids and vitamin and mineral content that wild and pastured animals have, which impacts how our cells function.

7. We eat a pale comparison of the amount of daily fiber that our earliest ancestors would have consumed. Fiber effectively cleans out and supports our bodies' natural detoxification processes.

Of course, it is not feasible for every human being in the modern world to resort to a hunter–gatherer lifestyle. Eating paleo today means eating a variety of vegetables, with a heavy emphasis on dark, leafy greens, as well as seeds, nuts, and sprouts, a smaller amount of fruits, and lean meat. Processed foods and grains are not permitted on the paleo diet. Nor is dairy.

Going "paleo" does not touch on the fact that our earliest ancestors also went for extended periods of food shortages sometimes, which forced periods of fasting, a topic I discuss more in the next section.

To summarize, eating paleo today means avoiding all grains—wheat, oats, barley, rye, rice, corn, millet, quinoa, and teff—dairy, refined sugars, and of course, processed foods and industrial animal products. What you will find in plenty on a paleo diet is lots of green leafy vegetables and herbs, as well as a large variety of other plant-based foods, such as fruits, roots and tubers, seed, and nuts, as well as lean pasture-raised meat, such as chicken, and seafood.

Paleo-Diet Off Limits:

1. Processed foods
2. Grains and flours
3. Dairy
4. Refined sugars (cane sugar, corn syrup, maple syrup)

Paleo-Diet Staples:

1. Green leafy vegetables and herbs
2. Roots, tubers, squashes and pumpkins, seeds, nuts, sprouts, legumes, fruits, berries, coconuts, avocadoes, olives, mushrooms, and so on: a wide variety of available plant foods
3. Pasture-raised (if at all possible) fresh meats and eggs
4. Fish and seafood, particularly small, cold-water fish, such as sardines and herring

5. For the occasional sweetener, small amounts of honey
6. Fresh water, herbal teas, fresh-pressed juices

A NEWER DEVELOPMENT: THE KETOGENIC DIET

The paleo diet is fresh, balanced, and rich in nutrients. It also encourages lots of raw veggies and fruits whenever possible. In raw form, fruits and veggies contain a full complement of vitamins and minerals, as well as enzymes that help to digest them more completely. Ideally, your food would also be organic or grown without pesticides and chemical fertilizers.

But for many people, the paleo diet may still be too high in foods that have what is called a high glycemic index—think sugar and starches. *Glycemic index* is the amount that a food may elevate blood glucose (sugar) levels. You may have also heard of the term *glycemic load,* which is slightly different from glycemic index. Glycemic load looks at the types of carbohydrates in addition to the *amount* that blood glucose levels may rise. A bowl of Cornflakes®, for instance, has a glycemic index of 81 and a glycemic load of 70.1, both high. This is so because Cornflakes® not only have sugar in them but also a lot of grain. A Mars® bar is 65 and 40.4, respectively, whereas a fresh yam is 37 and 8.4 respectively. Even though yams taste sweet and have a certain amount of natural sugar, they do not have grain-based carbs, which means the glycemic load is lower. From a diet perspective, then, the paleo diet may include foods that have a moderate glycemic index but a lower glycemic load than standard American fare due to the absence of grains. You may say, why is this important?

If a food's glycemic load is high, then, of course, the body will produce more insulin, and we've already discussed the chain of events that happens with high sugar–high insulin. You will recall also that cancer loves sugar. When blood sugar levels are high, any cancer cells in the body have an immediate fuel source. These factors are reason enough to lower sugar intake even more than when shifting to a paleo diet, particularly if you are struggling already with prostate disease, and especially if you have prostate cancer.

The ketogenic diet answers this need to slash sugar levels from our daily diet. The "keto diet" that has captured so much attention today can be traced to the 1920s when researchers at Harvard Medical School observed that children who suffered from epilepsy stopped having seizures during fasting. After 2–3 days of not eating, these children experienced marked improvement in seizure activity. What these researchers suggested was that the absence of food amounted to a sharp decline in carbohydrates, which forced the body to burn fat. Shortly after the Harvard team made their observations, a physician at the Mayo Clinic proposed that the metabolism benefits from fasting could be obtained if the diet produced ketones in the bloodstream.

The result was the ketogenic diet, a high fat, low carb, low protein diet. The word, ketogenic, means "ketone producing," and ketones are a by-product of breaking down fats in the body. When we fast, exercise strenuously, such as running a marathon, or are in a state of starvation, the body turns to fat stores for energy. When it does, "ketone bodies," or "ketones," are produced.

Those of us who were brought up on the USDA Food Pyramid may have a difficult time wrapping our heads around turning that pyramid upside down. Instead of eating a diet high in carbs and low in fats, the keto diet tells us to do exactly the opposite. What is also interesting about the keto diet, although researchers don't talk about this, is that it also falls in step with eating patterns of our ancient paleolithic ancestors who surely would have gone through periods of fasting during seasons when there was little plant food to gather. During these times, the likely mainstays of the diet would have been what they hunted or fished. The body has a built-in mechanism for doing without the immediate energy derived from sugar and carbs and turning instead to fat for energy.

Like the paleo diet, the keto diet does not permit any processed foods and grains, which are high in carbs. Sugar, even from fruits and honey is off-limits. Unlike the paleo diet, the keto diet says "no" also to roots and tubers, including yams, as well as winter squashes and fruits, with the exception of low-sugar berries occasionally, such as blackberries and raspberries. Also, unlike the paleo diet, the keto diet does permit dairy.

Keto-Diet Off Limits:

1. Processed foods
2. Grains and flours
3. Sugars and sweeteners
4. Root veggies, tubers, yams, and winter squashes
5. Fruits, except low-sugar berries occasionally

Keto-Diet Staples:

1. Green leafy vegetables and herbs
2. Seeds, nuts, sprouts, coconuts, avocadoes, olives, mushrooms, and so on: a wide variety of available plant foods
3. Pasture-raised (if at all possible) fresh meats and eggs
4. Fish and seafood, particularly small, cold-water fish, such sardines and herring
5. Dairy
6. Fresh water, herbal teas, fresh-pressed vegetable juices

By now, it should come as no surprise to you that I have a strong opinion about sugar and carbs. Shifting away from sugar and carbs is an essential step for preventing deterioration of the prostate, and, if you already have prostate disease, for getting it under control. If you have been diagnosed with prostate cancer, then I strongly encourage you to consider shifting to a keto diet, or better yet, the my Prostate-Specific Paleo-Keto Diet that I describe in the next section. In my view, you do not have much room to compromise if you have prostate disease and especially, prostate cancer.

BEN'S PROSTATE-SPECIFIC PALEO-KETO DIET

As I explained earlier, the nutrients in food are the building blocks of your body. If you were building a house, you would build it to be sturdy and withstand the test of time. If you were building your body by hand the way you might go about building a house, you would likely build it much the same way: to be sturdy and withstand the test of time.

It turns out that your body is building itself every day. It only makes sense to build with good materials. The diet that I introduce to you in this section provides you with those good materials.

Before getting into the details of my Prostate-Specific diet, I want to add a few suggestions here to build on what I have discussed already about paleo and keto. First, we need to return to the basics. This means eating food as close to its source as possible—that is, eating fresh foods. If you know a local farmer and/or have a farmer's market in your area, by all means, buy from them. If you can grow some of your own, by all means, do so. There is no fresher food. Whereas a head of lettuce from your local farmer may have been fresh-picked that morning, that same variety of lettuce in the supermarket may be a week old, traveling on average a good 1500 miles in the US from farmer, to warehouse, to supermarket, to you. Not only will your food be fresher when it is local, but you will also benefit from a more intimate relationship with it and your nutrition, which translates to being more intimate with your health.

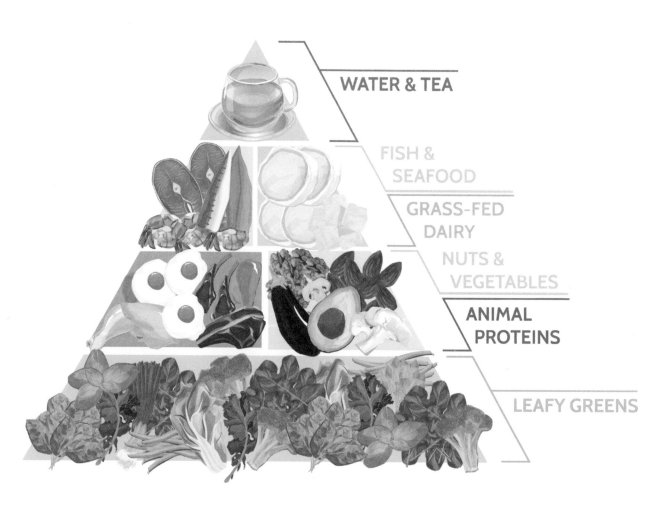

WATER & TEA

FISH & SEAFOOD

GRASS-FED DAIRY

NUTS & VEGETABLES

ANIMAL PROTEINS

LEAFY GREENS

Second, I encourage you to think of each meal as feeding your health. How often we go for comfort foods, but more often than not, these are the very foods that are wreaking havoc on our health: mac and cheese, mashed potatoes, French fries, grilled cheese, pizza. The list goes on. Every morsel of food that goes into your mouth is an opportunity to boost your health.

To explain Ben's Prostate Specific diet, I want to also explain what happens when carbs are our primary energy source compared to what happens when fat is our primary energy source. When carbs are broken down in the gut, they enter the bloodstream as glucose—sugar that the body can use. Once in the bloodstream, signals go out to the pancreas telling it to produce and release insulin. Now insulin is in the bloodstream to pick up the glucose and convert it into glycogen. Insulin also helps to send glycogen into muscle and liver cells where it will be stored for future energy needs.

Glycogen is the first source of energy called on when the body runs out of a fresh supply of glucose. The body does not rely only on glycogen for energy though. Once stores of glycogen are depleted, the body will turn to burning any available fat, either from what we have eaten recently or the fat stored in our body.

On a low-carb keto diet, the objective is to reduce the number of carbs you eat each day so that the body no longer relies on glycogen stores for energy. Instead, it turns to dietary and bodily stores of fat. Reducing to 20 grams of carbohydrates or fewer per day shifts the body into "ketosis," which, as you will recall, means the body starts to break down fatty acids and uses those for energy. Within two weeks of eating this way, the body becomes ketogenic.

Once ketosis is established, 35–40 grams of carbohydrates per day will maintain it, although some people can maintain ketosis at 50 grams of carbs. The carbs need to be replaced in the diet by healthy fats. When the body "learns" to burn fats instead of relying on glycogen for energy, it will begin to burn excess body fat too.

But there are other reasons making this switch makes sense. The amount of glycogen that your body can store is very limited compared to the amount of fat your body can store, even without being overweight. As a result, switching your primary source of fuel from carbs to fat gives you far more stamina. The most important benefit, of course, from a health standpoint, is the effect on insulin production. Lowering insulin production gives your pancreas a well-deserved rest and reduces the chances of becoming insulin resistant while also reducing the amount of inflammation-causing blood sugar.

My Prostate Specific diet is a modified and combined version of the best of both the paleo diet and the keto diet. It is grain-free and free also of root-vegetables and other sweet veggies and fruits. It is also dairy-free (unlike the keto diet). This diet encourages as many fresh foods as possible, and especially, lots of green leafy vegetables, nuts, seeds, and sprouts, herbs, meats and eggs from pastured animals, seafood, and healthy fats, such as the fats from coconuts and avocados.

Ben's Prostate Specific Diet Off Limits:

1. Processed foods
2. Grains and flours
3. Sugars and sweeteners
4. Root veggies, tubers, yams, and winter squashes
5. Fruits, except low-sugar berries occasionally

Ben's Prostate Specific Diet Staples:

1. Green leafy vegetables and herbs
2. Seeds, nuts, sprouts, coconuts, avocadoes, olives, mushrooms, and so on: a wide variety of available plant foods
3. Pasture-raised (if at all possible) fresh meats and eggs
4. Fish and seafood, particularly small, cold-water fish, such as sardines and herring
5. Dairy, ideally from organic grass-fed goats and cattle
6. Fresh water, herbal teas, fresh-pressed vegetable juices

Many people might describe such a diet as radical. Having my prostate cut out would be radical, to me, much more so than this diet. If you think about it, changing your diet to avoid all processed foods and industrially produced animal protein is not really radical by comparison. Getting rid of industrial foods is the most urgent change to make for your health. You may need to take the rest of the changes in gradual steps, reducing your carbs to the target level of 20 grams per day to reach ketosis. That said, you may feel that some of these suggestions are simply not in the cards for you.

Making changes on behalf of your health always needs to be manageable so that you can sustain them. Otherwise, you'll find yourself right back at the beginning and either giving up on these recommended changes or despairing that you can't do it right. There is no right or wrong here. There is only better. For many people, the process of shifting from SAD to my suggested Prostate-Specific diet needs to be a slow one. Remember that you are the boss of your health. Not me. Not anyone else. If you can get into the mindset of making every meal a fresh meal that feeds your health, then you are well on your way to taking your health into your own hands.

BEN'S BASICS FOR THE PROSTATE-SPECIFIC DIET

A simple rule of thumb for what your Prostate Specific meal should look like is this:

- Two thirds of the plate should be covered by leafy vegetables plus other veggies (with the exception of root veggies and winter squashes)
- One third of the plate should be reserved for protein and fats, such as that from fresh meat, fish, or eggs.

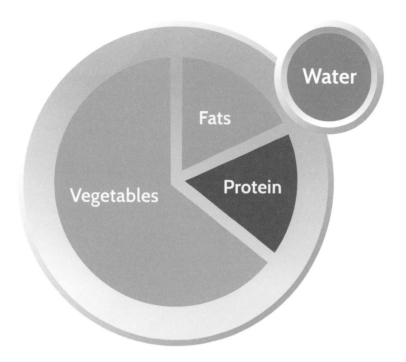

If you have an enlarged prostate only and your symptoms are minimal, then you have room for a little compromise—not so if you have prostate cancer.

If you need to make these diet shifts in phases, you might consider doing so as follows:

1. **Let go of all processed foods and industrial meat sources.** This won't be easy if you are like many people from the US and UK who are accustomed to convenience foods, but commit to this step, and it will make the rest of the diet program much easier to follow.
2. **Bypass the sugar.** This includes natural sweeteners like honey, maple syrup, and concentrated fruit juices.
3. **Massively cut back on dairy.** (only a small amount of grass fed dairy is acceptable, none if you are battling aggresive prostate cancer) It is essential that you not compromise on this one. I have devoted a whole section below to the dairy problem.
4. **Eat more veggies and eat more of them *raw*.** Have at least one green salad every day.
5. **Switch to grass-fed animal protein sources.** These meats are leaner, and they also contain a greater percentage of healthy omega-3 fats and vitamins and minerals.
6. **Go organic.** Eating organic means you don't have to worry about your food being contaminated with chemical pesticides, and if you buy from small organic growers, the produce is likely to be more nutrient-rich because even organic farming practices deplete the soil, particularly on large-scale organic farms.

Following these guidelines will improve your nutrition, support the "building blocks" of your cellular function, and give you the best chance at preventing or curing prostate disease through nutrition.

Let's summarize the Prostate-Specific Diet.

SAY YES! TO THESE FOODS:

Eat Your Greens and Other Veggies Too

In general, vegetables are the healthiest food you can eat, with no downside. In Western cuisine, more often than not, they are considered an accompaniment to the meat and grain portions of a meal. Try to make veggies the main event with some protein as an accompaniment. In other words, change the balance.

Eat your greens and veggies, and as often as possible, eat them raw. Raw vegetables preserve all the nutrients and enzymes that help to break them down during digestion. In other words, raw veggies come with a full complement of digestion aid. In raw form, the also contain "pre-biotics," which are the precursors that support probiotics and a healthy gut. Get creative with salads. It is amazing how much variety you can add to your diet by changing the simple green salad into a raw plate of plenty. You might also try juicing veggies, particularly if you want concentrated nutrients without the filling fiber.

Other methods include steaming, baking, roasting, and stir-frying them. Those methods of cooking preserve more of the nutrients and the flavor. Sous vide, a French term that means "under vacuum," as a newer method of preparing veggies (and meats too). With sous vide, you place the desired food into a glass jar and cook it in a water bath at a very low temperature (around 130–140 degrees F) for much longer than normal cooking times, anywhere from 1–7 hours, but up to 48 hours, depending on the food. The food cooks evenly throughout to a desired doneness. And since it is sealed in a jar inside the water bath, nutrients are not leached out and lost to the water. Many three-star Michelin restaurants now use the sous vide method.

Add Nuts, Seeds and Sprouts

With a diet that leans heavily toward fresh veggies, nuts and seeds are invaluable. Nuts, seeds, and sprouts are excellent sources of healthy fats, including omega-3 fatty acids, as well as protein, fat-soluble vitamins, minerals, and antioxidants. You might think of nuts and seeds as the storehouse of nutrients for the next generation of plants, and when we eat them, we benefit from that nutrient density. Walnuts and almonds are particularly nutritious because they contain high amounts of vitamin E, and walnuts are loaded with omega-3s.

Almond skins, along with the skins of many other seeds and nuts, contain phytic acid, which is hard to digest. It is a good idea to soak them overnight in filtered or mineral water so that they begin to germinate. In the morning, pinch off the skins, then place them on a cookie sheet at the oven's lowest temperature so that they dry out, which may take several hours.

The soaking process produces enzymes that break down the phytic acid and makes the nuts and seeds easier to digest.

Note that California legislation allows almonds to be sold as raw even if they have been irradiated or pasteurized by other means. This process, in effect, pre-cooks them, which kills the enzymes that break down the phytic acid. If at all possible, try not to eat California almonds. Try instead to get imported Italian almonds.

Natural seeds (not roasted) of all kinds can be beneficial, especially pumpkin, sesame, and sunflower. Also, try sprouts of various kinds, which you can get from a good health food store. Sprouts are simply seeds that have started to germinate. You can also sprout seeds in a glass jar at home. Many vegetable seeds can be sprouted: broccoli, radish, alfalfa, pumpkin, sunflower, and so on.

Eat "Alkaline" Foods for Long-term Health

Perhaps you have heard people talk about acid-producing foods and alkaline-producing foods. What are these foods? And what's all the buzz?

When foods are digested, the byproducts are in the forms of acids (pH < 7) and bases (pH > 7). A base is alkaline. The majority of SAD foods are acid forming, as are animal proteins, which means when these foods are digested in the body, there is an acid byproduct. When vegetables and fruits are digested, on the other hand, there is a base byproduct from the breakdown process. Most plant-based foods are alkalizing, therefore.

Many people eating standard American fare may be in a chronic state of low-grade "metabolic acidosis." The same is true for eating a diet high in animal protein, which can happen with paleo or keto eaters who overload on animal products without adding a large amount of fresh vegetables. There is a lot of debate about this topic and whether diet can cause metabolic acidosis, but many researchers say that, yes, over the long-term, it does. In other words, it's the long haul that is important, and you will recall from the beginning of this guide that prostate disease doesn't just come on suddenly. By the time prostate disease is detectable, a slow, steady process of decline has been years in the making.

If the researchers are right who say that dietary metabolic acidosis is a legitimate concern, then it's worth noting that a high "acid-load" diet—think, SAD diet—should be avoided. These researchers say that as soon as the body notes an acid imbalance, it begins immediately to rebalance. To do this, it pulls minerals from tissues, including muscles and bones. Studies have shown that a high acid-load can contribute to osteoporosis, the formation of kidney stones, and reduced muscle mass.

For people who are beginning to show signs of insulin resistance, this acid load can make things worse and even lead to diabetes. Some researchers say low-grade metabolic acidosis is also linked to high blood pressure, hormone imbalances, and chronic inflammation in the body. What makes matters worse is that as we age and our kidney function declines, the acid load from our diets can get worse.

In addition to foods that form acids during digestion, some foods also contain high levels of acid already. Coca-Cola®, for example, contains high levels of phosphoric acid. Phosphoric acid is a strong contributor to dietary acid load.

On the other hand, almost all veggies, herbs, nuts, seeds, and fruits are alkalizing foods. These foods contain high amounts of a variety of minerals that are base-forming in the body, including potassium and magnesium.

Even though there is not yet consensus on this matter, there is enough research to support the view that it's a concern for us to pay attention to it. What's more, the information on acid–base balance also falls in step with views about how our ancient ancestors ate. I think researchers have only recently touched the tip of the iceberg on this matter, and my advice it to take it seriously and look at the benefits of eating a plant-rich diet that is high in a variety of minerals. It certainly can't hurt!

Of course, it goes without saying at this point that changing what's on your plate also means cutting out all processed food and dairy. Making these dietary changes, and especially adding to lots of raw vegetables, nuts, and seeds, will go a long way in reversing metabolic acidosis and the problems that it causes.

Fruits Are High in Antioxidants

Many people following encouragement to eat more fresh foods resort to eating more fruits. But the nutrient content of fruits pales in comparison to that of vegetables. They have fewer vitamins and minerals than vegetables, with the most prominent being vitamin C. The largest component of fruit is water followed by rather too much sugar. Fruit does contain a healthy amount of fiber. Fruit has not always been as sweet as it is today. Because of our desire for increasingly sweet fruits to keep pace with all the other sweets we eat, however, growers increasingly cultivate fruits to have more and more sweetness. Fruit in moderation is a good part of a balanced Prostate Specific diet, unless you have insulin resistance or diabetes. As with vegetables, it is best to eat fruits raw, because they contain important enzymes that help with digesting them.

There are a handful of fruits that are strongly encouraged on the Prostate Specific diet because they are so high in antioxidants, healthy fats, and fat-soluble vitamins. These include low-sugar berries, such as blackberries, raspberries, and blueberries, as well as avocado. Acai and goji berries are a bit more exotic but very high in antioxidants, as are pomegranates.

Let's talk about antioxidants for a moment. We know that antioxidants are good for us, but what do they do? The process of using energy in our cells is "oxidative." You might think of it like passing gasoline through the engine of your car to drive it down the highway. The car has a combustion engine that burns fuel and blows by-products out the exhaust. A similar by-product process takes place in our cells. When we eat a diet high in plant foods, naturally occurring antioxidants "scavenge" these by-products of energy metabolism.

All of the environmental and chemical pollutants that we are exposed to on a daily basis also release "oxidants" into our bodies. Technically, these oxidants are called reactive oxidative species, or ROS, a term you might have heard before. ROS contribute to inflammation in the body, so understanding how not to add to ROS and what foods scavenge for them is important for supporting prostate health and reversing prostate disease.

Surely, hunter–gatherers were not thinking about antioxidants when they were foraging local plants! They also were not dealing with all of the processed foods that we eat today or the modern-day pollution in the air, on our clothes, and in our food and water. It is only in the past couple of decades that we've developed a strong interest in eating high antioxidant foods. And it is likely becoming clear by now how important it is to fill your plate with fresh, health-boosting plant-based foods: vegetables, herbs, nuts, seeds, sprouts, and fruits.

Fruits in moderation do provide important acid–base balancing minerals. Bananas, though high in sugar, have a much lower glycemic load than most grain-based foods, and they are loaded with potassium. Avocados are rich in healthy fat-soluble vitamins A and E. So, don't be caught in the belief that you have to avoid all fruits because of the sugar content. Simply enjoy them in moderation, and go for the lower sugar berries.

Lean Meats Are Rich in Nutrients

Enjoyed in moderation, lean meats are a beneficial part of the Prostate Specific diet, particularly when they are free-ranging chickens. Beware: industrial poultry facilities are no different from industrialized cattle agriculture. Because most people prefer "white" meat chicken over "dark" meat, these industrial facilities breed chickens and pump them full of growth hormones to be so disproportionate in breast size from normal that the majority of them cannot even stand up by the time they are slaughtered. They have higher fat content than chickens raised in pastures, and, like CAFO meats, the meat from industrial chickens contains residues of hormones and antibiotics. In the long term, eating the meats of these chickens can be harmful. It is best, therefore, to eat free-range chickens. The same is true for eggs. I discussed above the benefits of healthy farming practices on the meats, but I cannot emphasis enough the importance of understanding where our food comes from and how it is grown.

Eggs can be a well-balanced source of protein, again, when eaten in moderation: up to 3 eggs per day is fine.

Duck and goose are fine once or, at most, twice a week.

Fish Is an Excellent Source of Healthy Fats

Fish is an excellent source of lean animal protein. It is also high in rich omega-3 fatty acids, the healthiest of fats. Most animal protein on the Prostate Specific diet should come from fish or seafood. As I discussed above, what our food eats, we eat, so with the increasing amounts of pollution in the oceans, it is best to avoid large fish, such as tuna, salmon, and cod. These larger fish accumulate mercury, a heavy metal that now pollutes our seas. Environmental pollutants are also reason to avoid too much farmed-raised fish. Small fish like sardines, mackerel, and herring are still harmless, because their meat does not contain high levels of pollutants and are therefore good for you.

Fats are an essential nutrient. But not all fats are created equally. Saturated fats from grain-fattened animals, processed and refined hydrogenated oils, and trans fats all contribute to disease and are found in industrialized foods: meats from CAFO animals and cured meats, as well as processed and fried foods. Fats from nuts and seeds and fish support our health, and the proper ratio of omega fats is key.

Many nuts and seeds that are pressed and bottled into oil and used for cooking and dressing salads are high in omega-6 fatty acids. These include sunflower, safflower, and canola oils. Flax and chia seeds, as well as walnuts, on the other hand, are high in omega-3 fatty acids, as is seafood, particularly Antarctican krill.

A good ratio is 70/30 of omega-3 fatty acids to omega-6 fatty acids. Chances are, if the standard American diet is your mainstay, then you are more likely in the range of only 20–40% omega-3 with a substantial percentage of saturated and trans fats making up the rest. Omega-3 fatty acids are naturally anti-inflammatory and have been shown to reduce prostate cancer growth.

What about Plant Protein?

For the Prostate Specific diet, beans and lentils are a good source of plant-based protein, much like nuts. However, if you decide to do the ketogenic diet instead of the Prostate Specific diet though, you will want to avoid beans and lentils entirely since they contain starch, which converts to sugar in the blood rapidly. In that case nuts and seeds are good sources of keto-friendly protein.

Feed Your Gut

It is accepted widely now that the microbes living in our gut are an essential part of our health. The entire "community" of these organisms is called the "microbiome," and it consists of bacteria and other microorganisms that also live on our skin, in our mouths, and so on. The food we eat affects the types of organisms that grow in and on our body. Research has suggested that an altered microbiome may be linked to chronic inflammation.

Probiotic foods add healthy bacteria to our gut, but most of us think only of dairy yogurt when we think of adding probiotic foods to our diet, which won't do for the Prostate Specific diet. There are a host of other options. Fermented vegetables, like kraut and kim-chi are excellent sources of probiotic foods, and they are not that difficult to make. Many supermarkets, especially health food stores, now carry a variety of probiotic foods in their refrigerator sections.

Eat these foods in moderation:

Be Careful with Red Meat

You will recall that red meat from CAFO animals is fraught with problems: high saturated fat with low omega-3 fatty acids and minerals and laced with hormones and antibiotics. You will also recall that eating any animal protein contributes to "acid-load" in the body, putting us at risk for low-grade metabolic acidosis. Therefore, it is best to eat red meat sparingly, or better still not at all, unless you can get grass-fed, organically reared beef. It is also best to avoid char-grilled red meat and well-done steaks because burning meat generates carcinogens.

SAY NO TO THESE FOODS:

Processed Foods & Industrial Meats are a Danger

It should be clear by now that these foods do not support our health and contribute to prostate disease. If you do nothing else that I recommend in this guide, do this: cut out all processed foods, packaged and cured meats, and meats from animals raised on industrial feedlots. Making these changes will go a long way in preventing the further deterioration of your prostate.

Fried Foods Put You at Risk for Disease

The same is true for fried foods. It is fine to quick or "flash" stir-fry your vegetables for flavor, but putting them in a vat of hot oil is not. You certainly should not fry anything in breadcrumbs. The process of frying any carbohydrate, such as batter, breadcrumbs, or potatoes, creates acrylamides, which are known carcinogens. Also, heating most oils to the high temperatures needed for frying causes them to lose all beneficial enzymes and nutrients and worse still, break down into trans fats. Trans fats interfere with the ability of the body to absorb nutrients. So, if you eat trans fats you do not benefit from whatever else you are eating. Trans fats also are linked to atherosclerosis (hardening and blockages in arteries), which increases your chances of having a stroke or heart attack.

If you have to fry food on occasion use saturated fats, such as coconut oil, butter, lard, tallow, bacon drippings, palm oil, and avocado oil, or even goose fat. All of these have high smoking points and do not break down into trans fats when heated to high temperatures. Contrary to long-held views by the medical establishment in the West that saturated fats cause heart disease, there is actually no clinical data to support that contention.

Put a Stop to the Sugar!

I'm sure it is clear by now that avoiding sugar is critical for your health.

Apart from the issues I have discussed so far regarding blood sugar and insulin levels, as well as inflammation, there are other problems with sugar too. Sugar creates AGES (Advanced Glycation End Products), which line the inside of the arteries, contributing to plaque build-up, and causing them to lose their flexibility. Every time you eat sugar, therefore, you are putting yourself at risk for developing chronic disease.

The most common sugar substitutes are no solution either. They are just as bad as, if not worse, than sugar for men with prostate disease especially, because many sugar substitutes have cancer-causing agents in them. Honey, maple syrup, and concentrated fruit juices are, for the body, just another form of sugar. Stay clear of them. If you wish to sweeten food or you have a hankering for something sweet, turn to plain fruit, and in moderation.

I cannot emphasize this point enough: if you have cancer, the most important thing you can do to slow its development is cut out all sugar from your diet. Recall that cancer loves sugar.

Grain Is Not All It's Cracked Up to Be

For many years, I was persuaded that grain, particularly whole grain should be a staple part of a healthy diet. In fact, I was influenced by studies that showed how a vegan diet would improve prostate health. Research has since clarified that it is the addition and emphasis of vegetables, herbs, nuts, sprouts, and seeds, and not grain, that improves prostate health.

Eating a diet rich in whole grains did not work for me. I gained weight and continued to do so not matter what I did. Eventually, I even became officially diabetic. With all the grain, I was becoming increasingly insulin resistant. It was insulin resistance that caused my weight to climb continuously and eventually contribute to diabetes. I have since learned the term "breaditarian" for the way that many people eat who shift to vegetarian or vegan diets. Grains are filler foods, and they are high in glycemic load, which as I discussed above, can contribute insulin resistance.

After three months of being on a ketogenic diet, I lost 15 pounds and 6 inches around my waist. It was a ketogenic diet that finally allowed me to reduce my belly fat. Had someone told me years ago that switching to a diet reliant on fat for energy would help me to lose weight, I would have told them that was impossible. I would have insisted on a grain-based diet, but time and again, I have seen people struggle with body weight and insulin resistance on a grain-based diet.

✳ While I am now a proponent of the ketogenic diet, I see benefits of the paleo diet as well, so I have pulled from the best of both to create the Prostate Specific diet, which includes a few changes to both the paleo and keto diets to optimize prostate health. These changes include cutting out caffeine and dairy.

Caffeine

To date, research has not provided conclusive evidence about caffeine's impact on the development or worsening of prostate disease, including cancer. Some researchers suggest that a few of the chemical compounds in caffeine-containing tea and coffee may actually have anti-cancer properties. Others say caffeine may cause cell proliferation (increased in numbers and size) and hyperplasia (enlargement). Researchers consistently warn that caffeine irritates the symptoms of BPH, prostatitis, and prostate cancer. Men who drink caffeine tend to have worse symptoms of urinary leaking and waking in the night to pee than those who don't. The Prostate Specific diet strongly discourages drinking caffeine for these reasons.

Milk Does Not Do a Body Good

The Prostate Specific does not permit cow's dairy, with the exception of butter or ghee from pasture-raised (grass-fed) cows. There are good substitutes these days for non-dairy milk. Nut "mylks" are easy to make at home using a good blender. Almond mylk is one of the easiest. After sprouting them and pinching off the skins, soak the nuts in filtered or spring water over night, pour off the water, place the soft almonds in the blender, blend and add water in increments to the consistency you like. You may want to add a touch of vanilla for a natural sweetness without sugar or a tiny pinch of Himalayan sea-salt to balance the taste. Himalayan sea-salt has a varied mineral content most akin to the mineral content of our bodies. This almond mylk is quite rich. Hempseed mylk is another option and has the added advantage of providing the exact combination of amino acids to offer a high-quality protein.

It is clearly more work and effort to create your own nut or hempseed mylk than it is to buy a ready-made product. Many supermarkets carry an assortment of non-dairy mylks now. However, it is a good idea to always keep in mind that these products contain additives to keep them shelf-stable. Many also contain sugar, so if you buy ready-made nut mylks, make sure they are sugar-free and that they are not artificially sweetened. Also, manufacturers' priority is to maximize profit, which means that in an effort to lower their costs, they often use lower quality products, which are also less likely to be organic. The bottom line is that although it is more convenient to buy ready-made, you will never get the same quality as you do when making something yourself.

If you do not like the taste or texture of nut mylks, you might also try drink goat's milk. Many people tolerate this dairy quite well. Goat's milk has a composition that is entirely different from cow's milk. That said, many people are allergic to the proteins (casein and whey) in any form of dairy, so it is a good idea to go off all dairy completely for 4–6 weeks. Then try goat's milk and see how you feel. If you have any stomach cramping, nasal congestion/runny nose, itchy skin or rashes, or any unusual symptoms, it may be that your body can't process these proteins. If you can get raw, unpasteurized goat milk and other products, such as butter, yogurt, and cheese, you may find that you tolerate them quite well. In raw form, these dairy products contain the enzymes necessary to digest them—including the proteins I just mentioned that can be so troublesome.

A word of caution here: the most common milk substitute is soy milk. Soy milk is not a healthy substitute. Soy mimics estrogen. And estrogen, as you now know, contributes to prostate disease. Although soy has been consumed in the Eastern world for thousands of years, it is only eaten when it has been fermented, and even then, only as a condiment in relatively small quantities. The majority of soy produced in the US is from GMO crops, and we just don't know enough yet about the effects of GMO crops on our health. Even organically grown soy mimics estrogen, so it's best to avoid it. The same is true for soy-based cheeses and butters. Avoid them.

In fact, steer clear of all non-dairy butter spreads and margarines. None of them are healthy, despite the enthusiastic advertising. They are produced by pumping hydrogen through oil at a high temperature. This process is called "hydrogenation" and causes the formation of trans fats. Trans fats increase the risk of heart disease. They also block the absorption of good amino acids. As I said before, grass-fed butter and ghee, as well as goat butter, are fine. You might also try substituting organic, cold-pressed olive oil for butter.

Refined Vegetable Oils Are Not Your Friends

Once upon a time, before the advent of vegetable oils, people ate saturated fats rendered from cooked meats, typically lard and tallow, as well as butter and cream in their cooking. Heart disease wasn't an issue then. It was so rare, in fact, that family doctors were not accustomed to treating it.

The same is not true today, of course. Refined vegetable oils from corn, canola (rapeseed), safflowers, cottonseed, peanuts, and sunflower seeds, along with the explosion in sugar consumption, together have contributed to the many chronic diseases, including heart disease. The food industry, set on selling and making hefty profits on their products, conspired with researchers to say that cholesterol from animal fats was the culprit for the rise in heart disease. But these studies were distorted.

Cholesterol is not the issue. Things are always more complex than they seem. Cholesterol is actually necessary for the nervous and immune systems, and it helps the body defend against chronic inflammation.

The body actually makes cholesterol. Yet, an entire generation was force-fed the idea that low-fat, zero-cholesterol was the way to go to prevent heart disease. High carb/high sugar foods with refined vegetable oils became staples in the western diet. And the food industry raked in millions. There is plenty evidence now pointing to these food trends as a root cause of many of today's chronic diseases.

While saturated fats from grain-fattened cows are not encouraged as a mainstay of fats in the Prostate Specific diet, they are not the evil villain food marketers have made them out to be. The refined vegetable oils are worse. Organic, extra-virgin, cold-pressed olive oil and extra-virgin coconut oil are the only oils recommended on the Prostate Specific diet.

Here's what you need to know about refined vegetable oils, in a nutshell: they contribute to chronic inflammation. I emphasize the importance of reading labels carefully, especially in the US where labelling requirements are lax when it comes to the truth about extra-virgin and cold-pressed—which are the only unrefined oils, and the only oils you should eat. If possible, select extra-virgin, first cold-pressed olive oils from Italy. The truth is, these unrefined olive and coconut oils are not cheap. If there are cheaper ones on the shelves, they have probably been refined in some way. Don't buy them. Do yourself a favor and spend the money on the more expensive oil, even if it means using less of it at home. The test for good quality, unrefined coconut oil is that it should smell deliciously of fresh coconut. If it doesn't, it isn't what the label says it is. Obviously, you can't smell the oil from a sealed jar in the grocery store, but do look for "unrefined," "virgin," and "fresh-pressed" on the label. Then smell it when you get home. If it doesn't smell of fresh coconut, take it back and try another brand.

It is fine also to use butter from grass-fed, pasture-raised cows or butter from goats, and you can use animal fats and lard, providing again, that these drippings come from grass-fed, pastured animals.

More about Milk & Cow's Dairy

In the western world, milk from cows is promoted as a health food. You've heard it: "Milk, it does a body good." This is a marketing ploy that supports the dairy industry, not your health!

For decades, dairy advertising has been based on a false premise. The argument is that children need the calcium in milk to build strong bones and that adults need it to avoid osteoporosis. This claim is unfounded and is based on the dairy industry's interest in selling milk. We do not need milk to grow healthy bones and to keep our bones healthy. Instead, we need to stop eating the foods that take healthy minerals out of our bones, and if we follow a diet that is rich with plant foods and dark, green leafy vegetables, as well as healthy lean meats with rich bone broth added to the mix, we get all the minerals that our bones need.

Interestingly, the lowest incidence of osteoporosis is in countries that consume very little if any dairy. I'm referring to countries like China, Japan, and Thailand. The highest incidence of osteoporosis is in countries like the US and Britain where considerable quantities of dairy products are eaten. What is also interesting is that as Asian countries develop lifestyles and eating patterns similar to those in the West, the incidence of osteoporosis increases.

As if the message about the importance of dairy in a healthy diet isn't marketing ploy enough, the dairy industry also promotes a pastoral image of healthy cows munching contentedly on grass. Nothing could be further from the truth. Industrial dairy operations feed cows grain on feed-lots and line them up to industrial pumps in steel buildings to force their milk. Their living conditions are dreadful, much like the cattle feed-lots that produce beef. These conditions require antibiotics to stave off diseases.

Residues of antibiotics are in industrial dairy products. This means, when you consume conventional cow's milk, butter, or cheese, you are consuming a portion of the antibiotics given to them. There's more to this story and how practices of the modern dairy industry negatively impact your health.

Not many years ago, a typical milk cow produced a little more than 1.5 gallons of milk per day. Now that number is almost 14 gallons! That level of high production means that most cows have udders trailing along the ground. They get infected. As a result, almost all store-bought milk from industrial dairy operations contains trace amounts of blood, puss, and antibiotics.

Purely as a matter of economics, modern milk production keeps cows permanently pregnant in order to maximize milk production. Apart from the unnatural cruelty of exploiting animals in this way, there are implications for human health. Tests have shown that cows kept permanently pregnant have 200 times the normal concentration of female hormones in their milk, particularly estrogen. We know from my earlier discussion on estrogen that having an imbalance of female to male hormones can be detrimental to prostate health. Drinking milk containing a surplus of female hormones does just that.

This was not always the case. Before the need to keep cows in dairy production, farmers would stop milking pregnant cows. Not true today, and the further into pregnancy a cow is, the more estrogen her milk contains.

Milk also contains a natural growth factor, IGF-I, designed by nature to stimulate growth. But since milk is intended by nature for the mother's offspring, IGF-I in cow's milk is intended for growth and development of a calf, not a mature adult human. IGF-I signals cells to grow, and IGF-I of cows is identical to IGF-I in humans. Normal, healthy adult cells will ignore IGF-I. But cancer cells are not normal, and with IGF-I in the mix, they accept the signal and begin to grow more rapidly. In other words, IGF-I stimulates cancerous growth.

There's more still! Milk also contains two proteins that I mentioned before, casein and whey. Experiments feeding casein to mice with prostate cancer showed an exponential explosion of growth in their cancer compared to those not fed casein. Finally, some studies suggest that dairy may contribute to insulin resistance. Despite having a relatively low glycemic load, dairy products are considered to be highly "insulinotropic," which means they cause insulin spikes, perhaps as much as does white bread. The bottom line is that dairy is very problematic for prostate health. I strongly encourage you to make it a priority to delete it from your diet.

Why Prostate Disease is Less Prevalent in East Asia

As with osteoporosis, in countries like China, Japan, and Thailand, the incidence of prostate cancer is a tiny fraction of that in western countries. In fact, once upon a time, prostate disease was so rare in China that a doctor might never see a case in his lifetime.

Dr. Jane Plant, an epidemiologist, whom I mentioned in the Introduction, looked at these differences when she was diagnosed with breast cancer. After the fifth recurrence and metastasis (spreading) of cancer and multiple bouts of surgery, chemotherapy, and radiation, Dr. Plant was told that she was at an end stage and would die. At this point, already knowing of the significant differences in the incidence of breast cancer between East and West, Dr. Plant decided to start trying to figure out why.

She noticed that the difference was most likely due to the fact that the diet of the East (specifically, China, Thailand, and Japan) contains far fewer animal fats and virtually no dairy products. This discovery set her on a course of investigating milk and what it might contain that could contribute to higher incidences of breast cancer in the West. She also stopped eating any food that had even a trace of dairy. Her tumors began to shrink immediately. Within six weeks, she was able to show—to the complete astonishment of her doctors—that a large tumor that had bulged from the side of her neck had completely disappeared. Eventually, all her tumors disappeared, and after fifteen years of a strictly dairy-free diet, she had no further recurrence of cancer, at all.

You may be wondering what Dr. Plant's story has to do with prostate disease. Table 1.1 shows a similar picture to what she discovered about breast cancer. The rates of prostate cancer in the UK and US are far greater than those of the Asian countries. The data also show that when ethnic Chinese become American citizens and they and their families adopt more of a standard American diet, the incidence of prostate cancer increases. Why is this?

The difference in consumption of dairy seems to make a substantial difference. While eating trends are changing in China due to Western influence, the average person in China consumed about 12 pounds of dairy per year in 2003. The average American, on the other hand, consumes around 276 pounds of dairy a year. This difference is staggering and worthy of attention, particularly given the differences in the incidence of prostate disease.

TABLE 1.1

	COUNTRY	PROSTATE CANCER IN MALES
CHINA	China, Qidong country (rural)	0.5
	China, Shanghai (urban)	2.3
	China, Tiajin (urban)	1.9
	Hong Kong	7.9
JAPAN	Japan, Hiroshima	10.9
	Japan, Miyagi	9.0
	Japan, Nagasaki	9.1
	Japan, Osaka	6.8
	Japan, Saka	6.7
	Japan, Yamagata	7.9
WESTERN	England & Wales	28.0
	Scotland	31.2
	USA (Caucasian)	100.8
	USA (African American)	137.0

Table 1.2 shows a later analysis. It's a little hard to compare with the previous data in Table 1.1 because of differences in the population grouping and the means of collecting and standardizing that data. We can see, nonetheless, how the incidence of prostate cancer and mortality are far higher in the western group as a whole than the eastern one. These figures tell us that prostate disease is not inevitable. They also suggest pretty convincingly that there is a strong link between diet and prostate disease.

TABLE 1.2

COUNTRY	INCIDENCE OF PROSTATE CANCER	MORTALITY
China	1.7	1.0
Thailand	4.5	2.9
Korea (South)	7.6	2.8
Japan	12.6	5.7
New Zealand	100.9	20.3
Australia	76.0	17.7
Canada	78.2	16.6
UK	52.2	17.9
USA	124.8	15.8
Iceland	81.0	23.0

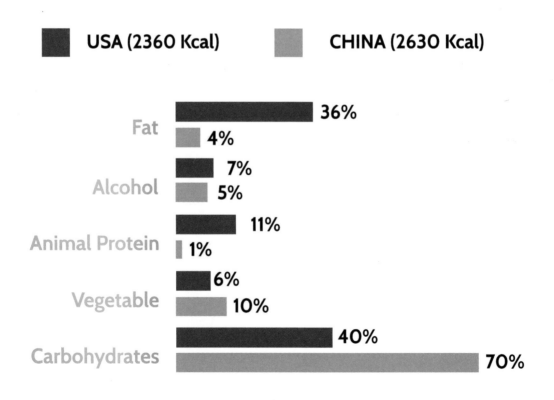

USA (2360 Kcal)   CHINA (2630 Kcal)

	USA	CHINA
Fat	36%	4%
Alcohol	7%	5%
Animal Protein	11%	1%
Vegetable	6%	10%
Carbohydrates	40%	70%

WHY EAT ORGANIC?

Most people understand that industrially produced vegetables contain pesticides and other synthetic pollutants. But they may not understand why these pollutants are significant for human health. I want to shed light on that here.

The body has mechanisms for dealing with what it sees as foreign substances and mounts an immune response to any non-food substance that makes its way in. All synthetic chemicals are in that category of "foreign substance," which the body registers as threatening. This ongoing response to danger puts the immune system on chronic alert. We have discussed already that when the immune system picks up the signal that there is a problem, it mounts an inflammatory response to repair the damage and rid the body of the perceived threat. When that inflammatory response is acute, it is healing, but when it is chronic, it can lead to disease. Consuming foods that have been sprayed with chemical pollutants can, over time, cause low-grade chronic inflammation, and potentially, disease. Anything you can do to avoid this situation in the body will be a boost to your prostate health.

Also, however well the body deals with toxins, it cannot rid itself of all of them. It filters them through the liver, and if it can't filter all of these toxins out at once, the body stores them in other parts of the body, much like it does excess energy. Whereas excess energy is stored in liver and muscles, excess toxins are stored in fat and other organs that are hormone-dependent. Some of these toxins mimic hormones, and we have seen already that consuming products that mimic hormones can trigger problems in the prostate.

These toxins are also linked to cancer. Cancer rates have increased exponentially over the past handful of decades. There is reason to believe that agricultural and industrial toxins are a causal link.

As Shown in table 1.3 Plants Seem to be much better "farmers" than we are. As a result of their clever "gardening" for millions of years, we humans have inherited many feet of beautiful fruitful topsoil all around the globe with zillions of happy mircoorganisms thriving in it. In their best-selling book, Secrets of the Soil, Peter Tompkins and Christoper Bird state that, "the combined weight of all the microbial cells on earth is twenty-five times that of its animal life; every acre of well-cultivated land contains up to half a ton of thriving microorganisms, and a ton of eathworms which can daily excrete a ton of humic casings".

TABLE 1.3

Organic Produce vs Conventional Produce

	% of dry weight		Milleequivalents per 100 grams dry weight					Trace amounts per million dry matter			
	Total Mineral Ash	Phophorous	Calcium	Magnesium	Potassium	Sodium	Total Mineral Ash	Phophorous	Calcium	Magnesium	Potassium
Snap Beans *Organic*	10.45	0.36	40.5	60.0	99.7	8.6	73.0	60.0	227.0	69.0	0.26
Commercial	4.04	0.22	15.5	14.8	29.1	0.9	10.0	2.0	10.0	3.0	0.00
Cabbage *Organic*	10.38	0.38	60.0	43.6	148.3	20.4	42.0	13.0	94.0	48.0	0.15
Commercial	6.12	0.18	17.5	13.6	33.7	0.8	7.0	2.0	20.0	0.4	0.00
Lettuce *Organic*	24.48	0.43	71.0	49.3	176.5	12.2	37.0	169.0	516.0	60.0	0.19
Commercial	7.01	0.22	16.0	13.1	53.7	0.0	6.0	1.0	9.0	3.0	0.00
Tomatoes *Organic*	14.20	0.35	23.0	59.2	148.3	6.5	36.0	68.0	1938.0	53.0	0.63
Commercial	6.07	0.16	4.5	4.5	58.8	0.0	3.0	1.0	1.0	0.0	0.00
Spinach *Organic*	28.56	0.52	96.0	203.9	237.0	69.5	88.0	117.0	1584.0	32.0	0.25
Commercial	12.38	0.27	47.5	46.9	84.6	0.0	12.0	1.0	49.0	0.30	0.20

SOIL, MICROBES AND PROSTATE HEALTH

Industrial agriculture depletes the soil. It does so via erosion of fields laying fallow, intense planting and harvesting of row crops, and use of chemical pesticides. As a result, vital nutrients that would otherwise make their way into the plant are lost, and microbes that work in tandem to support healthy plants are wiped out. Conventional produce is lacking in essential nutrients and microbes that feed our gut. The result? Vegetables and fruits that may look pretty but have a paltry nutritional value compared to plant foods grown even 50 years ago.

A big difference between industrial and organic agriculture is that industrial agriculture focuses on the crop and on weeding out any pests (insects, weeds, fungi) that might threaten the crops. This approach relies on chemicals to fertilize the plants with the few essential minerals plants need in order to grow and produce, and chemicals to ward off anything that might threaten the crop. Organic farmers, on the other hand, focus on growing the soil, believing that healthy soil feeds healthy plants. Organic growers also recognize that to grow soil, they need to make sure the microbes are healthy.

This difference in approach to growing makes its way to the table. When foods are lacking, our bodies don't get the full complement of nutrients needed to grow, function, be healthy, and ward off disease. The pesticides that wipe out soil microbes and plant "pests," our bodies also wipe out the healthy microbes in our gut.

It is only recently that researchers have begun to grasp how important a healthy microbiome is for the healthy functioning of all our body systems. It helps to "educate" the immunological system, and when this community of microbes is in disarray, chronic inflammation may occur. What is important to note here is that the chemicals sprayed on plants may have a link to prostate cancer by the fact that they disrupt our microbiome.

There's more to this chemicals-on-plants story. The microbiome also has a role in affecting hormone levels. When the microbiome is out of whack, hormone balances of estrogen and testosterone can be thrown off, and we've discussed this impact already too. Here, we see a link between industrial agriculture and prostate disease contributing to systemic inflammation and hormone imbalances. Of course, researchers are just beginning to explore these complex links, but I am here to tell you that eating organic whenever possible is not only important for the health of your prostate, doing so will keep those foods that may actually cause disease out of your daily diet.

SALVESTROLS: ANOTHER REASON TO EAT ORGANIC

In the early 2000s, researchers identified a class of phytonutrients (plant nutrients), which they termed Salvestrols. Salvestrols are a plant-based cousin to the cholesterols found in animals. They protect plants from fungi. Grapes, for instance, are predisposed to "blight," but Salvestrols have a natural anti-fungal property that protects their skins from fungus. In plants, Salvestrols serve, in some ways, like our immune system. They are found in many red and green plants and herbs, and of those we eat, red grapes, tangerines, and strawberries, particularly.

It turns out that cancer cells contain an enzyme that healthy cells do not. When we eat Salvestrol-containing foods, this cancer-cell specific enzyme activates the Salvestrols, which then produce byproducts that are, in turn, toxic to the cancer cells. They destroy the cancer cells. Salvestrols are a food-based mechanism to abolish cancer cells without damaging healthy cells! For a long time, scientists have suggested that our bodies produce cancer cells daily. A healthy immune system, along with phyto-nutrients, such as Salvestrols, abolish these cancer cells right away.

Produce raised by industrial methods has minimal if any Salvestrols. Industrial agriculture, through use of antifungal sprays, as well as through the development of new varieties of plants, has reduced the levels of Salvestrols substantially. Older "heirloom" varieties of plants that are grown organically would naturally have the highest amounts of Salvestrols. Hence, eating organic produce enhances the level of cancer-destroying Salvestrols that we consume.

INTERMITTENT FASTING

Calorie restriction and intermittent fasting have been the topic of research debate since the 1930s. Over the past decade, with rates of obesity and chronic diseases on the increase worldwide, interest in alternate day fasting (ADF) programs has followed suit. Research shows that calorie restriction by ADF or restricting the number of hours per day that a person eats is linked to increased life span, reduced age-related diseases, including cancer, as well as reduced obesity and type-2 diabetes. Researchers are not clear yet about why this is so, but some suggest that it has to do with lower levels of IGF-1.

You may remember from the section on dairy that IGF-1 is related to cell growth, which runs rampant in cancer cells. Intermittent fasting can reduce IGF-1 by up to 75%, thereby reducing cancer cell activity. There is also evidence to suggest that intermittent fasting reduces systemic inflammation and helps to balance hormones. For these reasons, I strongly encourage a program of intermittent fasting as a part of my Prostate Specific diet program.

There are two ways to go about intermittent fasting. The first is to limit the number of hours per day that you eat. You might gradually delay your first meal of the day to later and later in the morning, while also making your final meal of the day earlier. Ideally, you would limit "eating period" to 8–10 hours in every 24, say from 10 or even 11am to 7pm on a daily basis. You will find that your body will gradually adjust to this eating schedule, particularly since you will not be relying on carbs for energy. If you find that you are struggling to keep to the fast, check to make sure that you are getting a healthy balance of fats and not relying on carbs for energy, which should become less and less of a problem as you adopt my Prostate Specific diet.

The second way to go about intermittent fasting is ADF. For 1 or 2 days every week, reduce your calorie intake to 20% or 25% of what you normally eat. If you normally eat 2000 calories per day, your fasting days would be limited to 400–500 calories. Many people gradually lower this fasting amount to only water on fasting days.

ALternate day Fasting

There are instances in which intermittent fasting is not recommended. For people with type-1 diabetes, or women who are pregnant or nursing, or persons with eating disorders, intermittent fasting is not recommended. Doing so may significantly compromise your health or that of your fetus or infant in the case of pregnant and nursing women, respectively. But for most men interested in restoring overall health and that of theprostate, I strongly encourage that you give it a try.

LOSING WEIGHT

Obesity is the largest single cause of disease in the Western world. Being overweight does increase your chance of getting prostate cancer, among other cancers, as well as diabetes, heart disease, and many of the chronic diseases that plague people in the modern world. These dietary changes that I have recommended often result in weight loss. Normalizing your weight, if you happen to be overweight, will support your overall health. If you choose to follow the Prostate Specific diet program that I have outlined, you will no longer be eating the foods that spike insulin, cause excess energy to be stored in your body and toxins in your cells, and that throw your hormone balance out of whack.

Intermittent fasting, however you choose to go about it, may also contribute to weight loss. In whatever ways you decide to go about these diet changes that I recommend, you certainly are likely to feel better. And you can rest in knowing that you are restoring your health.

A FINAL WORD ON DIET CHANGES

Making dietary changes can be a challenge. We have ingrained habits about eating that are not only related to what the food industry and agriculture are dishing out. We also have emotional ties to certain food habits, family traditions, and social pressures that can make it difficult to start and stick with a new way of eating. My suggestion is to get familiar with my Prostate Specific diet. Look again at what needs to go and what you want to add more of. Then take it one step at a time. If you remember to make health priority #1 and to make every meal one that feeds your health, you will be well on your way to making the Prostate Specific diet a new habit. Increasingly, it will become a welcomed part of your daily routine. Most importantly, be kind to yourself when you go off course—because everyone does on occasion, particularly in the beginning—and simply get back on track.

LIFESTYLE: THE MODERN TOO MUCH

Earlier in this chapter, I discussed how our modern, rushed lives have changed the way we eat. I emphasized that the majority of us lean toward convenience foods because we are so busy and that all too frequently we sit in front of a screen to eat. There's a lot more to this story of our modern lives that is impacting our health.

I also said that 70% of all diseases now are considered to be chronic diseases, prostate disease included. In developed countries like the US and UK, communicable diseases, such as cholera, are no longer the major source of illness and death, which they were in the 18th and 19th centuries and before. Rather, with the advent of vaccines and antibiotics, as well as water and food hygiene, most of us are more likely to suffer from diseases of "too much." We eat too many empty-calorie foods, are typically too stressed by the hurried pace and demands of our lives and too overloaded with environmental pollutants.

The effects of all this "too much" is that it overloads our body's natural capacities to stay healthy. Most of us don't realize that our body has a natural inclination to be healthy. Because conventional medicine is focused on treating disease, we, like our doctors, tend to think about what might go wrong. Many of us take for granted that our body has all the functions it needs to be healthy and ward off disease naturally.

You may be thinking, then why are so many people sick with one problem or another? It's the "too much" issue. If we want to be healthy, we need to look at our modern lifestyle. Now, I'm not saying we need to turn back the hands of time to a fantasied human time that was easier or disease-free. Human history has always faced challenges unique to the times. And thanks to modern medicine, many of the diseases of the past are no longer an issue for most of us living in the modern world. Of course, there are plenty of people in developing countries for which that is not true. For the majority of us living in the modern world, the issue of disease today is largely one of "too much."

I have discussed at length the "too much" issue related to our SAD way of eating. Here, I want to talk about "too stressed" and "too overloaded." All three of these issues add up and stress our body's threshold for coping.

"TOO STRESSED"

It doesn't take much imagination to understand what I mean when I say, "too stressed." Most of us can immediately feel it in our chest, throat, neck, or the area just below our breast bone. Think, for a minute, about your average week or your average day. How much time do you spend commuting to and from work? How much time do you spend stressing about completing everything that needs your attention every day? How much of your day is spent racing from one place or task to another? How many hours do you spend worrying about money, family responsibilities, caring for an elderly parent, a sick child, or a struggling partner or friend? How much "free-time" do you spend ingesting the onslaught of news, 99% of it increasingly bad? How much of that free-time is spent scrolling through social media feeds? And how much of what shows up on the screen leaves you feeling a little less enlivened than before you started to scroll?

Even trying to fit into our day the things we do to take care of our health can become stressful in the face of "not enough time." As impossible as it may seem, we can get out of this stress rut. For the good of our health, we must.

Every time our body is alerted to some kind of stressor we move into fight–flight–freeze mode—be that stressor a car that stops short in front of us, the sudden realization that we clicked "reply all" to an email chain when we intended to respond privately to just one person, or news of a mass shooting halfway across the world. I talked in the section on the paleolithic diet about how our biology has not caught up with culture when it comes to what and how we eat. The same is true about how our body responds to stressful events. No matter what the stressor, our biology perceives it as a potential threat to our lives, and a complex cascade of reactions takes place in the body to protect us from harm. These reactions speed up the heartrate, increase blood pressure, make us more alert, and at the same time, shut down the body's restorative processes that function during eating and sleeping.

Fight–flight¬–freeze keeps us safe in the face of harm in the immediate circumstances (like running from a tiger!). Over the long-term, however, or when stress just keeps adding up, this stress-response mode takes a toll on the body. Those same reactions that make us alert in the face of danger release hormones and chemicals in the body that over the long haul trigger inflammation, challenge the immune system, and cause "wear and tear." In other words, in the short-term, our body copes effectively with threats. But without physically discharging it (fighting or running from a wooly beast!), our coping functions start to take a toll on the body, and in time, on our health.

The reality is that we can't avoid all the stressors of modern life, but we can do a lot to lessen our exposure and mediate our response. We can be judicious about how much time we spend in front of a screen. We can try to simplify our lives by reading books, for instance, instead of staying glued to the onslaught of input from our screens. The next time you turn on the TV or any streaming device, make note of the violence, (even on comedy programs!) that we are becoming increasingly desensitized to psychologically. Our bodies still register it though, and it is contributing to disease.

We can also slow down. How much of the rush and hurry is real? Pay attention to what really needs attention today and what can wait. Our culture rewards us for being productive, efficient, and multi-tasking. Put a halt to that madness! Plenty of studies show that multi-tasking does little more than contribute to our stress and potentially put us in harm's way, because our attention is too fragmented. Make "extra time" where you tend otherwise to rush. For instance, you might leave a few minutes earlier for work and walk if you live in an urban area. Take breaks during the day to catch a breath of fresh air. Eat your meals in silence or with friends and family, but not in front of a screen. By all means, try to notice when you are rushing, and put the brakes on.

Make time also for play. What do you enjoy doing to relax? Make time for these activities that restore you. And get outdoors, if possible. The amount of research showing the benefits of being outdoors and/or in nature is growing exponentially. Take a walk in a park if you live in an urban area, or enjoy an hour- or day-long hike if you have access to trails. Not only does the body's stress response calm in natural environments, but it also quiets as a result of moving.

You might also take up practices, such as Tai Chi, yoga, and mindfulness-based-stress-reduction, or other mindfulness practices, all of which calm the mind and the body. A growing body of research shows that these practices actually change how our genes are expressed from one moment to the next, potentially correcting a gene mistake bent toward cancer. The promise of this type of change is that it may effectively stop cancer before it starts. These stress-reducing practices also reduce the other stress response chain reactions, such as systemic inflammation.

Most importantly, don't let stress define your life. You've heard the saying, "Choose your battles." The same is true for stress. Start choosing how to manage the stressors that are going to come up inevitably.

"TOO OVERLOADED"

There are now tens of thousands of synthetic chemicals in our environment that have never been tested adequately as to their effects on human bodies. What's more, these chemicals are increasing in numbers so rapidly that it would be well-nigh impossible at this point to test them with any measure of satisfaction. By chemicals, I'm referring, of course, to the overwhelming numbers of factory and agricultural agents, but also chemicals that have become a taken-for-granted part of our daily lives: cleaning and laundering agents, cosmetics and body-care products, textile and clothing sprays, and countless chemicals used in construction materials, like paints and glues in particle board, for example. Even if every single chemical newly introduced into our environment were rigorously tested, the problem of environmental pollutants would not be solved.

It is no longer a matter of testing individual chemicals. There are so many now, and they interact with one another in the environment, on our cloths, and in our homes and offices. There is virtually no way of assessing the cumulative effect of all these chemicals together. And we can't even fathom the long-term consequences on our health of these agents.

In a very real sense, we are like goldfish in a bowl unable to escape from the largest chemical experiment ever performed. To make matters worse, every chemical and pharmaceutical known to humans has been making its way into the water supply since we first started manufacturing them. What's really worrisome is that water treatment facilities increasingly recycle sewer water back into drinking water—after cleansing, of course. But these cleansing methods leave not only traces of every chemical out there in our drinking water, they also dump disinfectants into our water. Chlorine is the primary disinfectant, but there are others too.

What are the effects of chronic exposure to all these chemicals and the reactions between them? We really don't know the extent of the impact they are having on our health. What we do know is that many of these chemicals disrupt and wreak havoc on our endocrine (hormone) system, contributing to a host of hormone-related diseases, as well as fertility issues, genetic birth defects, breast cancer, liver cancer, and prostate disease, to name just a few.

Also, the disinfectants the water treatment facilities use disrupt the balance of healthy microbes in our microbiome. This disinfectant effect from tap water has an effect similar to that of pesticides on plants: kills healthy bacteria living in our gut and the rest of our body. And, of course, the trace amounts of antibiotics, chemo-therapy agents, and other pharmaceuticals challenge and weaken our immune system. Municipal water facilities cannot filter out all of these chemical agents draining into our water system. The water that comes out of the tap is a far cry from the pre-Industrial age, pristine clean waters that were alive with minerals from surface waters rushing over the earth. But that's a soapbox I'd best not jump on and digress!

There is one last kind of pollutant I want to discuss before moving on to talk about what we can do to protect ourselves, and that is the automotive and industry-generated air pollution—the source of smog in our cities. It also includes smoke from cigarettes—first, second, or third-hand. First-hand cigarette smoke is derived from smoking directly. Second-hand smoke is derived from being within breathing distance of a person smoking. And third-hand smoke is that which settles into a person's clothes or sits stagnant in a smoker's home or cars. All these forms of smoke are linked to cancer.

Automotive and industry-generated air pollution and cigarette smoke contribute to "oxidative stress," which I discussed in the section on fruits and the health benefits of antioxidants. Oxidative stress is linked to inflammation and negative effects on genetic expression. In other words, it can switch on factors that affect how new cells are expressed, and may switch on factors that generate cancer cells. Oxidative stress can also accelerate aging. Anything that contributes to systemic inflammation or that is linked to cancer should be avoided when it comes to keeping your prostate healthy.

What can you do about being overloaded with these poisons? First, get rid of all household cleaning and laundry agents that are not natural and/or are perfumed. By natural, I mean, organic, plant-based, products that are "eco-friendly." By perfumed, I mean any scent that does not come from essential oils. Laundry detergents and dryer sheets are the worst offenders. Get rid of all perfumed laundering agents. Instead of dryer sheets, you might try wool dryer balls to fluff your laundry. This new cleaning plan includes removing all chlorine-based cleaning products from your household. There are highly effective natural disinfectants and laundry brighteners that will not tax your immune and endocrine systems. And for problems, such as clogged drains, there are strong enzyme-based products to replace chemicals, such as Drano®.

Second, throw away all synthetic, chemical-based skin- and hair-care products and cosmetics. This includes synthetic antiperspirants, shaving products, and perfumes. As with cleaning agents, you will find a growing variety of grooming products that are natural. If you want scented products, make certain the scents are from essential oils.

Speaking of scents, say goodbye to all the room sprays, car scents, scented candles, and so on that "deodorize" and leave "smelling fresh" your home, office, and cars. These scented products are as bad as scented dryer sheets for your health. Burn unscented bees wax candles, which have a natural honey scent. Deodorize with vinegar and baking soda. You can also make your own room spray using 8–10 drops of lavender essential oil with a half to one cup of water. Not only does this spray not tax your immune system, but it also has a naturally calming effect on the nervous system.

It is best to drink filtered water. There are good under-counter water filtration systems that are much less expensive than whole-house filtration systems. If you drink bottled water, drink only spring water, and avoid plastic bottles. The plastic leaches chemicals that mimic estrogen.

Finally, it may seem obvious, but if you smoke, do yourself a favor and start a smoking-cessation program. If you live with someone who smokes, ask them to smoke outside and avoid breathing near them while they smoke. Try to avoid smoke-filled rooms or places where "third-hand" smoke may have settled. And if you live in an urban area, you might try avoiding walking or exercising outdoors along corridors with heavy traffic during commuting hours. Step away from the pump while gassing up your car, and consider keeping your windows closed in heavily congested areas.

THE BODY'S COPING THRESHOLD

All these lifestyle stressors of "too much" and "too overloaded" add up over time. Eventually, they tax the body's threshold for coping effectively. When they do, things begin to go awry with the body's natural functions. This breakdown in healthy functioning is the beginning of the long path toward chronic disease. Fortunately, the body is very forgivable because what it does best is tend to being healthy. This means that while we can't avoid all these stressors of our modern lifestyle, we can work with the body to support its natural inclination toward health.

I've made some suggestions here about changes you can make to minimize the impact of modern stressors, but there are two things I have yet to say on the matter. The first is a repeat of a point I made at the beginning of Part 2, which is the importance of taking your life into your own hands. When you begin to make health priority # 1, you may find that what at first seemed daunting now becomes increasingly easier and second-hand. By making these changes, your prostate will thank you, and you will feel better overall, gradually gaining energy and stamina, and generalized well-being.

The second suggestion is that it is important to understand that to be healthy, the body needs time to restore itself. Rest is essential. This includes adequate and good, sound sleep. It also includes giving yourself more time to just do nothing: to rest, restore, chill-out, and take it easy. It is during times of rest that the body rebuilds itself. It cannot do so when we are constantly on the move, rushing from place to place and task to task. Giving your body time to restore helps to dial it back from that "coping threshold" that is the point where healthy functions start to go awry. So, give yourself permission to take it easy—routinely.

There is more about modern life that's putting wear and tear on our bodies and contributing to chronic disease—and to prostate disease, no less. By and large, those of us living in the modern world have become increasingly sedentary. Whereas now we are encouraged to get a minimum of 30 minutes of moderate to vigorous physical activity every day, our ancestors of 40,000 years ago would have walked or run no less than 10 times that much in a single day! That's 5 hours, at least, of walking, running, and other physical movements, which our bodies are still biologically programmed to do.

In discussing the idea that our bodies have not caught up with our modern culture, we also need to factor in how sedentary we have become, at home and at work. Since 1960, the number of sedentary professions in the US increased by more than 20%. Tasks that even a generation ago required human effort are powered increasingly by machines. Technology is rapidly changing how we live. Convenience is the order of the day. And given that all living creatures are genetically programmed to conserve energy, most people are not inclined to be any more physically active than necessary, unless motivated to do so.

But our bodies are a bit of a contradiction, because while biology wants to conserve energy, we are also genetically programmed to move, which, of course, requires energy. Our bodies need to be active in order to be healthy. This is a simple point, but it's not a minor one. Getting into motion is a matter of preventing and healing disease!

A sedentary lifestyle is linked not only to expanding waistlines in developed countries over the past 50+ years. It is also a part of the chronic diseases picture. Now research is suggesting that long hours of uninterrupted sitting and physical inactivity may be linked to diseases of the prostate. If staying healthy and preventing disease is not motivation enough to get into motion, then perhaps the healthy benefits of physical activity for recovering from prostate disease will get the more slothful amongst us moving again. Rigorous physical activity is even linked to a decreased risk of advanced or lethal prostate cancer.

Let's be honest though. Shifting from being inactive to active can take some doing. For many of us, the idea of exercise (a word I have intentionally chosen not to use until now!) sends us running . . . to the TV. It's hard to get motivated to exercise when we've been inactive. And it's even harder when time seems so limited that we wonder where in the world we'll fit something else into our schedules. Sure, we know we need to move, but geez, it's one more thing to add to an already full and exhausting day.

NATURAL APPROACHES

MOVING LONGEVITY

Let's talk about what I mean by being physically active as a shift away from being sedentary. Obviously, everyone reading this guide can't just quit your jobs and embark on a life of physical labor. Nor would you want to. And not everyone is into sports. But there are changes you can make that will get you moving and positively impact your health.

Scientists use a term, "metabolic equivalent task," or MET, to measure the amount of energy you use during one minute of a task or activity. While lying down at rest, when the body expends the least amount of energy, MET is 1. When sitting at your desk or reclining on the sofa watching television, your MET is a little less than 1.5. It's about 2 when standing still. So, while standing desks have become a new trend marketed to improve health, it's not the increase in MET that these desks are providing. It's the reduced strain on the spine that comes from sitting. If you hit the deck and throw down two dozen push-ups—now you're talking about some physical activity! MET shifts to about 8, if not more.

The latest research tells us that frequent movement breaks for just a few minutes at a time will have a significant effect on overall daily MET. Taking a break every 20 minutes or so to get up and walk around your office for a few minutes, or doing a few calisthenics will go a long way. Who knows? Maybe you'll set a new trend in the office!

It's also important to . . . yes . . . get daily exercise, if you really want to prevent or heal disease. By exercise, I am referring to moderate to vigorous walking, running, cycling or other activities that keep your heart rate up, strengthening exercises that build muscle, and stretching to encourage flexibility. Without exercise, muscle mass diminishes significantly as we age, which affects our metabolism, the strength of our bones, and the effectiveness of our heart and blood vessels to pump fresh blood throughout our bodies.

BENEFITS OF EXERCISE

There are other benefits to exercise as well. Regular exercise . . .

- Supports a positive mood and outlook
- Improves prostate and sexual health by stimulating the production of testosterone
- Boosts metabolism, which helps support a healthy weight
- Improves sensitivity to insulin
- Preserves youthfulness by stimulating the production of growth hormone
- Reduces the risk of bone fractures by the strengthening effect of muscles pulling on bones
- Intervenes on systemic inflammation processes
- Decreases the risk of disease by strengthening the immune system

If you have prostate cancer, regular exercise has been shown to reduce PSA levels and decrease the risk of the cancer getting worse and spreading. Some studies have gone so far as to suggest that a regular moderate to vigorous exercise program may have effects akin to those of conventional medical therapies. I'm not surprised by this conclusion so much as I am by the fact that doctors are reporting it. Finally, for men who do choose to undergo conventional medical treatments, such as hormone replacement therapy, exercise has been shown to improve overall quality-of-life.

AEROBIC EXERCISE

Aerobic exercise is any continuous movement that gets your heart pumping. Typically, aerobic exercise consists of brisk walking, power walking, jogging, cycling, or swimming. But there are other forms of aerobic exercise that people enjoy, including cross country skiing—if you happen to live in a climate cold enough to do this regularly—and some forms of dancing. The American Heart Association recommends at least 30 minutes of aerobic exercise at least 5 days per week. If you are just starting an aerobic exercise program, it is best to consult your physician first if you have any type of heart condition or vascular disease.

Aerobic exercise can be moderate or vigorous. The American Heart Association considers moderate aerobic exercise to be, generally, any sustained exercise that keeps the heart beating at 50–70% of your maximum heart rate, and vigorous activity to be a sustained heart rate of 70–85% of maximum. This percentage of maximum heart rate is called your "target heart rate zone."

A general guide for determining your maximum heart rate is to subtract your age from 220. If you are 50 years old, your maximum heart rate is: 220 – 50 = 170.

Exercising moderately for 30 minutes, you would target a heart rate zone of 85–119 beats per minute for the entire 30 minutes or longer that you exercise.

Exercising vigorously for 30 minutes, you would target a heart rate zone of 120–144 during the exercise session.

You can track this heart rate zone by wearing a heart rate monitor or by taking your pulse. When taking your pulse during exercise, it is best to feel for your wrist pulse, not the pulse at your neck, and to count for only 10 seconds, because while you are counting, you likely have slowed your pace, and your pulse slows in turn. Multiply the number of heart beats counted during 10 seconds by 6 to get your beats per minute.

Here is an example. Let's say I am walking briskly for 30 minutes as a 50-year-old man, and I want to reach a moderate target heart rate zone of 85–119. After setting my pace, I notice that my breathing rate and volume has increased. To take my pulse, I may need to slow down just a bit to walk and be safe! I count 18 beats during those 10 seconds. Now I multiply: 18 X 6 = 108. I'm in my moderate heart rate target zone! Had the number been, say, 11 or 12, I would need to pick up my pace to achieve the minimum of 85 for my target zone.

I notice also how much I am exerting myself to keep this pace. This exertion is called "perceived exertion," and I use it as a measure of how to stay apace my target heart rate zone for the time that I am exercising. The same is true for achieving a vigorous target heart rate zone.

"Interval training" is a way to intensify aerobic without necessarily increasing the amount of exercise time. With interval training, you alternate between short bursts (about 30 seconds) of intense activity and longer intervals (1 to 3 minutes) of less intense activity during your 30-minutes of aerobic exercise. If you are in good shape, you might alternate between 30 second bursts of jogging with 1 to 3-minute intervals of brisk walking.

If you are just starting an aerobic exercise program, you want to approach interval training more easily and carefully. In this case, you might alternate between 30-second bursts of brisk walking and 1 to 3-minute intervals of leisurely walking. As you become more fit, you can certainly increase the intensity of each of the intervals, but the general idea of interval training is alternating intervals of intense with less intense activity.

Once you notice an increase in your stamina, you can begin increasing the intensity of the training. Whereas with conventional aerobic training, you would increase the time or effort of the entire exercise period, with interval training, you simply increase the level of effort without necessarily increasing the amount of time. In fact, with interval training, you don't need to exercise for as long as with regular aerobic exercise to appreciate the same benefits. Usually twenty to thirty minutes will suffice.

Part of the beauty of interval training is the flexibility with how you go about it. You might build up to 1-minute bursts and shorten the intervals of lesser intensity so that you eventually even out the intense bursts with the lesser intensity intervals across the entire exercise session.

What are the benefits of interval training? As with regular aerobic exercise, interval training improves your cardiorespiratory (heart and lungs) function, which means it also increases the amount of blood pumping through your body. And more blood flow equals more oxygen, which means cells have a key ingredient for the energy centers (mitochondria) to do their job. You'll feel a boost in energy and stamina as a result.

Interval training also lowers resting heart rate because the heart muscle gets stronger and pumps more efficiently. It requires fewer beats to pump the same amount of blood through the body. Blood pressure drops as well. Other benefits include improved levels of HDLs (high density lipoproteins—the good cholesterol) and better metabolism, which helps to control weight and reduce body fat. Interval training is a good way to bypass the "middle-age-spread." Finally, interval training sidesteps the boredom that can happen with an exercise routine that is the same day in and day out, which means you are more likely to keep it up over the long haul.

CALISTHENICS

Calisthenics is the term for repetitive exercises that use the weight and resistance of your own body to build strength and improve flexibility. By building muscle mass, calisthenics improve your metabolism and burn fat. There is some suggestion that they even improve the flexibility of the arteries, because, like interval training, these exercises rely on bursts of energy followed by periods of less intense activity. These intense–less intense waves mimic the natural flow of pulsing in the arteries and help keep them flexible as we age.

For the same reasons, calisthenics also improve the functioning of your heart muscle and lungs. Many people also feel a boost to self-esteem when they start to regain the strength of their youth—or even better it! By putting the body through a wide range of motions, calisthenics also improves flexibility.

Some studies suggest that acute, intense exercise, like calisthenics, positively impacts cancer. The idea behind this theory is that these bursts of intense exercise affect a whole chain of reactions in our immune system, endocrine system, and also inside cells. Exercise shifts the balance of proteins and enzymes that cancer cells rely on to grow. And, as I offered earlier in this section, these shifts may prevent cancer from worsening or becoming lethal.

Another great benefit of calisthenics is that they do not require expensive equipment. You can do them anywhere that you have floor space and a good 10 minutes of free time. The maneuvers are simple, instinctive, and easy to learn.

As with all exercise, it is important to begin a calisthenics program slowly. Below, I offer a list of calisthenics to get you started. If you do these exercises consistently, you can expect to see results in just a few weeks. In general, you should repeat each exercise as many times as you can, ideally building up to at least 30 times per exercise. You do not have to do all the exercises each day. Like interval training, a calisthenics exercise program gives you the flexibility to shake up your routine.

As a general rule, to build strength, you want to work the big muscles first. Your biggest muscles are the quadriceps on the front of your thigh followed by the hamstrings group on the back of your thigh. Like all muscles, even these big muscles lose strength if you don't challenge them. For any exercise, make sure you do the exertion part of the exercise on an exhale. And for the exercises below, see if you can start with 5 repetitions, gradually increasing as your strength improves.

ALTERNATING LUNGES

Benefits:

Alternating Lunges not only work the large quadriceps (front of thigh) and hamstrings (back of thigh) muscles, but they also engage the muscles in your core (abdomen, low back, and hips). Strengthening all these large muscle groups is a great way to prevent or reduce low back pain, improve posture, increase metabolism, and therefore burn excess energy and fat.

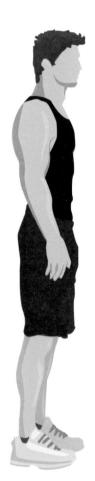
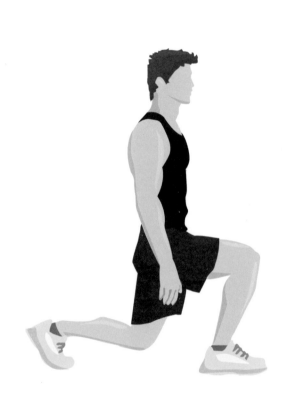

Instructions:

Stand tall, with your toes facing forward and your feet spaced approximately shoulder-width apart. Focus on a spot on the floor that is about 3 feet in front of your body. Begin by taking a few deep breaths. Then, when you are ready, as you exhale, carefully step your right foot out to the 3-foot spot in front of you. Inhale, then as you exhale, push off the ground with your right foot and come back to the starting position. Now, perform the same move with the opposite leg.

Safety:

Make sure your stepping foot is faces forward. Ideally, that knee should be bent at a right angle with your thigh, which should be parallel to the ground.

SQUATS

Benefits:

...the human body can do. When squatting you are
..., then you stand back up. Done correctly, squats
...out. Like lunges, squats involve large muscle groups
...strings, gluts (buttocks muscles), and (abs) abdominal
...ilar benefits as lunges and are fantastic for increasing

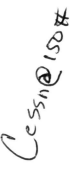

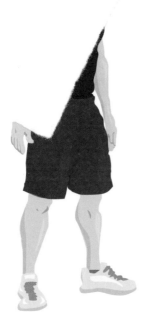

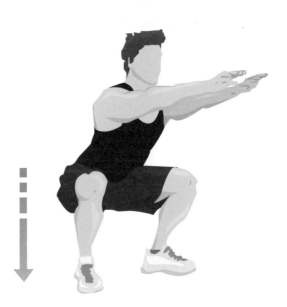

Instructions:

With your feet shoulder-width apart and pointing slightly away (about 15 degrees) from each
other, move your buttocks down and backward as if you are about to sit on a low stool.

The key is to keep your knees from extending beyond your toes. Keep your back straight.

It's best not to squat with your heels raised. If you are unable to keep your feet flat on
the floor, or do not initially have sufficient strength to squat, you can use a wall to support
your weight. Slide down the wall as if to sit, then slide back up.

Safety:

Turning your feet slightly outward helps the knees to track in a normal direction, preventing
knee injury and strain. To avoid any strain on the ligaments of the knee, you want your knee
cap to move in the direction that is directly in line with your second toe.

PUSH UPS

Benefits:

Perhaps one of the easiest exercise movements, the standard push up activates nearly every muscle in your upper body and core. Major muscles, such as biceps (front of arm), triceps (back of arm), pectoralis (chest muscles), deltoids (shoulder) and core muscles are activated to support your body while stabilizing your movements. Classified as a compound exercise, meaning multiple muscle groups are called upon to complete the motion, push-ups help train muscles throughout your entire body.

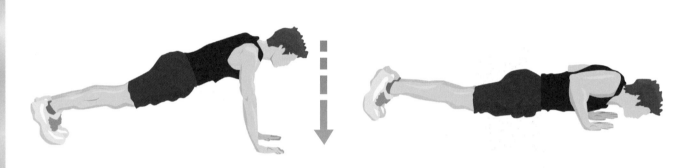

Instructions:

Place your hands firmly on the ground, and at a comfortable angle from the shoulders—not directly under them. Tuck your shoulder blades down, as if to slide them into your back pockets. Ground your toes into the floor to stabilize your lower half.

Brace your core, engage glutes and hamstrings, and flatten your back so that your entire body is neutral and straight. As you exhale, begin to lower your body, keeping your back flat and the neck in a neutral position until your chest reaches the level of your elbows. This end position makes a 45-degree angle between your elbows and the floor, and your upper arms are now parallel to the floor. Keeping your core engaged, inhale, then on an exhale push back to the starting position.

If starting push-ups in this way is too difficult, try the modified version with your knees touching the floor until your core muscle and arm strength improves to advance to the full-body push-up.

Safety:

If you do not give your hands a wide enough angle from your shoulders, or if you dip too low, you are at risk of developing a shoulder injury. Make sure to find that "just right" distance for your hands to be at a comfortable angle from your shoulders and to tuck your shoulder blades. Doing so engages your rotator cuff muscles, which support the shoulder joint and also protect these small, injury prone muscles.

ARM HAULERS (Superman)

Benefits:

Arm haulers are great for strengthening your back as well as the shoulder muscles. With increased back strength, will you find that your posture will improve, giving you a straighter and more confident stature. Also, day-to-day tasks/activities will be easier to perform because of the extra power you gain from this exercise.

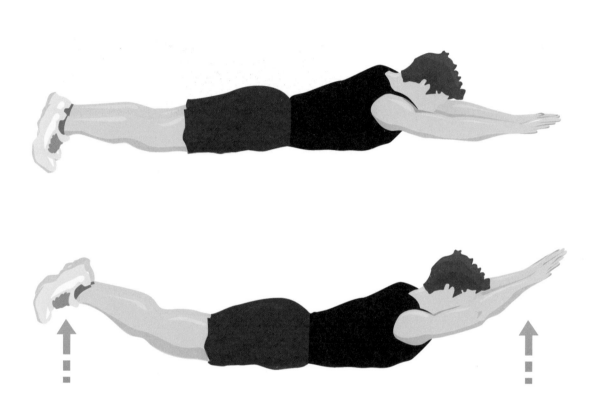

Instructions:

Arm haulers are an ideal exercise to do while recovering from push-ups.

Stretch your arms in front of you and raise your arms and heels off the floor holding the pose for 1–2 seconds then relax.

Safety:

This exercise is pretty straightforward and usually doesn't have risk of injury. It is a good idea to keep your feet shoulder-width apart to help you balance when you lift your heels from the floor.

PLANK

Benefits:

Arm haulers are great for strengthening your back as well as the shoulder muscles. With increased back strength, will you find that your posture will improve, giving you a straighter and more confident stature. Also, day-to-day tasks/activities will be easier to perform because of the extra power you gain from this exercise.

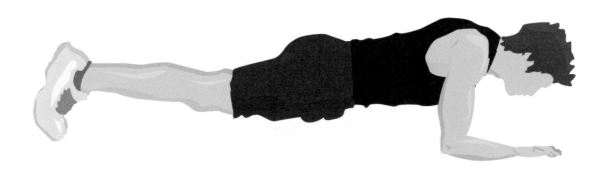

Instructions:

Get into push-up position on the floor. But this time, place your hands directly under your shoulders. Tuck your shoulder blades as with push-ups. Dip to the 90-degree angle that is the lower position of a push-up. Your elbows will be at your sides. Hold. Start with 30-second holds and increase to up to 2 minutes.

If this way of starting is too difficult, then try this modified version: place your elbows on the floor with forearms straight out in front, palms facing down. Elbows should be at a 90-degree angle with the shoulders. Tuck your toes and push your heels away from your body. Lift your body to form a straight plank between your shoulders and heels. Hold as above.

Be sure to breathe fully while also trying to relax when it becomes physically challenging.

Safety:

As with push-ups, you want to protect your shoulder with plank. You can do so by making sure to tuck your shoulder blades toward your back pockets and by keeping your elbows at 90-degrees. Do not dip below that.

PULL- UPS

Benefits:

Pull-ups, also known as chin-ups, are a simple exercise that are beneficial even if you can only do one repetition. Focusing on the back muscles, forearms, and biceps, pull-ups can quickly build upper-body strength and muscular tone.

You do need a pull-up bar to do this exercise, but they are easy to find and usually pretty inexpensive.

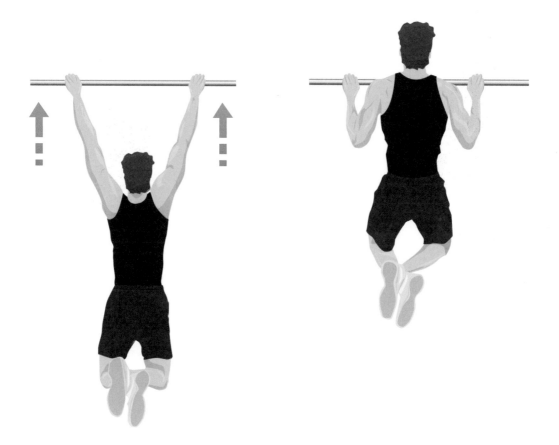

Instructions:

With basic pull-ups, palms facing away from you, pull your body up to bring your chin to the level of the bar. You can vary the width of your grip on the bar to work different muscles in your shoulders and back.

You can also change your grip to palm facing you. This way of doing the exercise is a little easier to do.

Safety:

Make sure the bar is securely in place and in a location that can support your weight before beginning this exercise.

DIPS

Benefits:

Like push-ups, dips are a compound exercise. Because multiple major muscle groups are involved, you build strength and tone in all of them by doing just this one exercise. Compound exercises also closely mimic movements that you perform in day-to-day activities, making them easier as you gain strength.

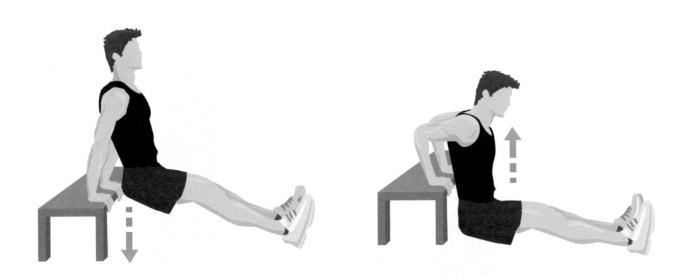

Instructions:

To perform dips, you need two parallel bars or desks that will hold the weight of your body as you dip between them. While putting one hand on each bar or object, lift your feet off the ground and cross one foot over the other; on an exhale, slowly lower yourself until your elbows are at about a 90-degree angle. Pause, inhale, then on your next exhale, push back up slowly.

If you don't have parallel bars of sturdy objects to hold your weight, you might try chair dips. Simply face away from the chair's seat, sit down on the edge of the seat and place your hands behind your hips. Your hands should be on the edge of the seat and shoulder width apart. Now on an exhale dip to a 90-degree angle at your elbows. Pause with the inhale, then on your next exhale, push back up slowly.

Safety:

To protect your shoulder, be careful that your elbows don't bend to an angle greater than 90 degrees. Doing so will strain the muscles on the front of the shoulder and the shoulder capsule around the joint.

CRUNCHES

Benefits:

As a core-training exercise, abdominal crunches help strengthen your abdominal muscles, which are crucial for good posture and balance. A healthy posture also helps prevent lower back pain and muscle injury.

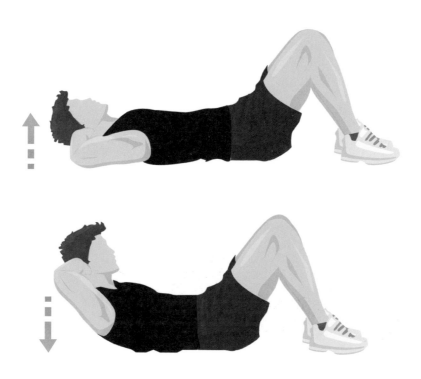

Instructions:

Lie flat on your back with your feet flat on the ground about hip-width apart, or with your knees bent at a 90-degree angle in relation to your spine (as if you are sitting in a chair while lying on the floor).

Now place your hands lightly on either side of your head, keeping your elbows in without locking in your fingers. Inhale. On the exhale, lift your head, leading with your chin and "crunch" your abdominals to shorten the distance between your chin and your pelvis. Hold for 1–2 seconds. On the next exhale, lower slowly back to the starting position and repeat for the second rep.

Safety:

With this exercise, you want to make sure to protect your neck. When the abdominals are weak, the tendency is to pull the head up no matter what. Lightly placing your hands on either side of your head without interlocking the fingers will avoid this tendency. You may not be able to 'crunch' very much in the beginning. With practice, the abdominals will strengthen and the tendency to pull on the head with the hands will decrease. Until then, make sure that you are not doing that!

LEG LEVERS

Benefits:

Leg Levers are an excellent exercise for the core, particularly for the lower abdominal area. Some people may regard this abdominal exercise as slightly more difficult than others, but you will build core strength very quickly with little repetition.

Leg levers are a favorite among many athletes who wish to train their core at an intermediate/advanced level.

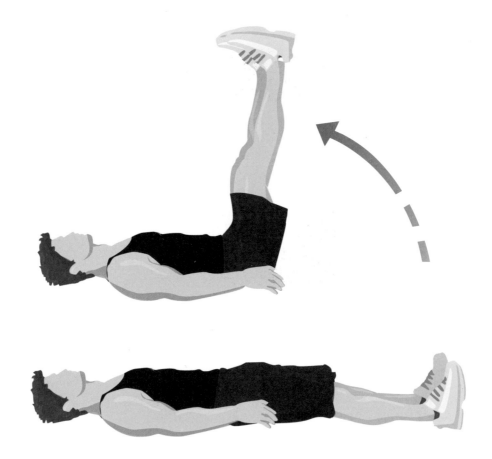

Instructions:

Lie on your back with your arms by your side, palms down, press the small of your back into the floor. Now lift your outstretched legs until they are in a vertical position—perpendicular with the floor and your spine. Inhale. On the exhale, slowly lower your legs back to the ground.

Safety:

To protect your back during this exercise, make sure that you press the small of your back into the floor and hold it there. Also, make sure that the exertion parts of the exercise (lifting and lowering your legs) takes place on an exhale.

ABDOMINAL FLUTTER KICKS

Benefits:

Abdominal flutter kicks target your abdominal muscles, and, like leg levers, the emphasize the lower abdominal muscles. They are also a superb workout for your hip flexors, where you will feel the effect as you increase the number of repetitions. Your middle and upper abs will also feel stimulation from this exercise, and you will get a great overall workout.

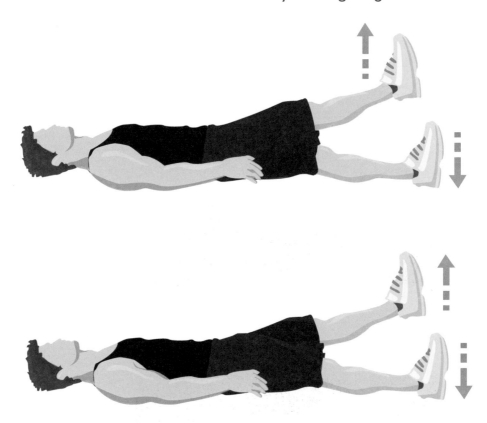

Instructions:

Lie on your back with your arms by your side, palms down, press the small of your back into the floor. Alternate lifting each leg from the starting position to about two or three feet off the ground. As one leg lifts, the other goes back to the starting position on the floor.

It is a similar motion to the one involved in swimming, only while lying on your back.

To advance this exercise, keep the lower leg 3-4 inches off the floor instead of returning completely to the floor.

Safety:

To protect your back during this exercise, make sure that you press the small of your back into the floor and hold it there. Also, make sure that the exertion parts of the exercise (lifting and lowering your legs) takes place on an exhale.

SCISSORS

Benefits:

Scissors are a great exercise for flexibility and general core strength.

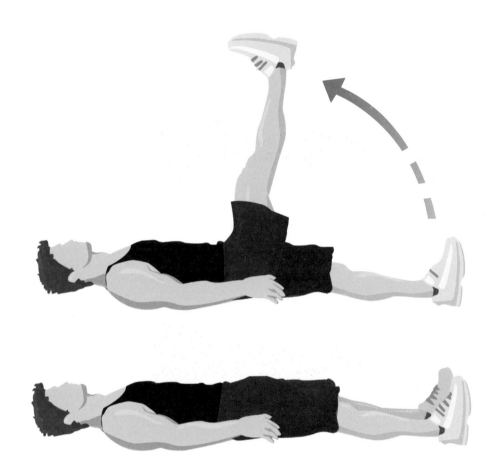

Instructions:

Lie on your back with your arms by your side, palms down, press the small of your back into the floor. The legs should be outstretched. On an exhale, lift both legs 3–4 inches off the floor, heels pressed out and away from the body. Now on an exhale, move your right foot toward the ceiling, which, when it is there creates an upside-down T of your body. Keep the left foot steady several inches off the floor. Pause. Now return the right foot to parallel with the left. On a next exhale, lift the left leg as you just did with the right. Pause. Then return it to the "start" position.

Safety:

As with the other abdominal exercises, you can protect your back by making sure to press the small of the back into the floor and keep it there during the exercise.

CALF RAISES

Benefits:

Calf raises strengthen your calf muscles and improve balance. Strengthening your calf muscles gives you more power to step forward, particularly when climbing hills on uneven terrain. Calf raises also help pump blood from your legs back to your heart. This is particularly helpful for long periods of sitting when blood tends to pool in the lower legs and feet, especially as we age.

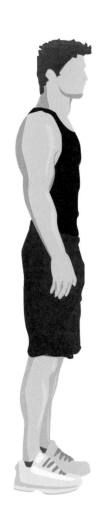 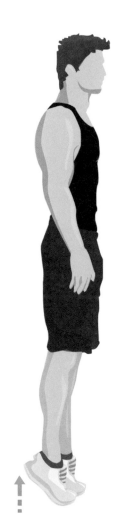

Instructions:

Stand with your torso upright, feet shoulder width apart. Raise the heels off the floor as you exhale. Hold. Then lower slowly back to the floor

You can increase the intensity of this exercise by doing it with dumbbells in hand.

Safety:

Calf raises are pretty straightforward and safe, generally speaking.

STRETCHING

As we age, we lose flexibility. Our tissues are prone to become more rigid, not just our muscles, but our tendons and ligaments as well. A regular stretching routine will help us stay injury-free, by improving joint range of motion and connective-tissue flexibility. Stretching also has a naturally calming effect, helping you to feel more relaxed. For this reason, many people incorporate a gentle stretching program into the evening, before bedtime.

We have already discussed the stress of our modern lives. Stress causes the muscles to contract and stay that way in a holding position. This stressful "holding" in our muscles creates a feedback cycle that creates more and more tension in the muscles and the mind. The tension can create pain eventually, leading to more tension. Stretching helps to break this cycle and ease the body and mind.

Stretching, like strengthening, can also improve posture, by breaking the tension-holding patterns in our muscles. A body more at ease and more upright plays a significant role in overall confidence as well. When our posture is more in alignment with how our bodies were originally shaped, less energy is spent on sitting and standing upright. Stretching actually makes sitting at our desks or walking easier.

And the improved blood flow to muscles, tendons, ligaments, and joints means the body can perform tasks for longer periods of time. This improvement in stamina reduces the likelihood of muscular fatigue and protects the body from injury, particularly if your work requires repetitive tasks. Even typing on a keyboard is a repetitive task that can result in injury.

Stretching also strengthens bones. By pulling and twisting soft tissues, which attach to bones, the activity of stretching tugs at them and makes them more pliable. This bone pliability is increasingly important as we age.

Specifically for prostate disease and particularly, prostate cancer, the calming effects of a gentle stretching program translate directly to improved functioning of our immune system. A growing body of literature shows that calming practices, such as yoga and Tai Chi, have immediate positive effects on the immune system, as well as how genes are expressed—two systems that are crucial for preventing and healing cancer.

The remarkable thing about stretching is that it is very easy to do, takes very little time and interruption from our daily tasks, and has immediate calming effects on our state of mind. To avoid injury when stretching, there are some general recommendations to follow. First, move into any stretch slowly, paying attention to the point when you begin to feel the stretch. Avoid "bouncing," which can tear micro-fibers of muscles and tendons. Finally, it is a good rule-of-thumb to find that sweet spot in a stretch that is about 60% of a maximum stretch. At 60%, your breath should be easy and soft, not tight as if holding on. This allows the body to relax fully into the stretch—which is not a "no pain-no gain" endeavor. You will also notice that once in the stretch, the intensity will diminish, and you can then move more deeply into it, but still with no more intensity than the original 60%.

QUAD PULL

Benefits:

Quad pulls stretch the (quadriceps) muscles on the front of the thigh, including the hip flexors, which get tight when sitting for long periods.

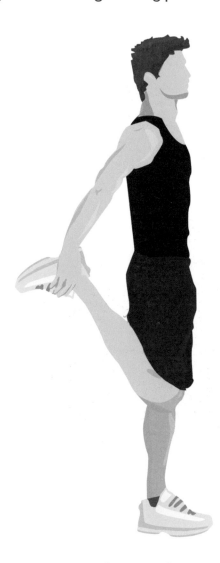

Instructions:

While standing on your left food, bend your right knee back and grab hold of your foot with your right hand behind your hips. Pull gently until you feel the thigh muscles beginning to stretch. Allow your breath to be soft and easy, holding the stretch for about half a minute. Release. Do the same on the opposite leg.

Safety:

This is a standing exercise. In the beginning, you may prefer to use a chair or wall for support, at least until you get more comfortable with the exercise. Once you find that you don't need the wall, you may want to do this stretch free-standing, which also has the benefit of exercising your balance.

TRICEPS PULL

Benefits:

Triceps pulls stretch your triceps muscles on the back of your arm.

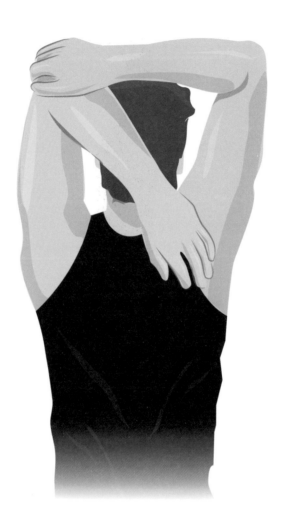

Instructions:

Stand with your feet shoulder width apart. Now put your right hand over your right shoulder and down toward the middle of your back. With your left hand, grab your right elbow. Take a deep breath, and on the exhale push your right hand down the middle of your back until you feel a good stretch on the triceps and bottom of the shoulder. Hold this pose for about half a minute, relaxing the breath. You can deepen this stretch as the muscle tissues give way and you begin to feel a release of initial tightness.

Safety:

If you feel any pinching in your shoulder or tingling in your hands or fingers, back off the stretch until these symptoms subside.

COBRA

Benefits:

Cobra stretches your abdominal muscles and keeps the spine supple.

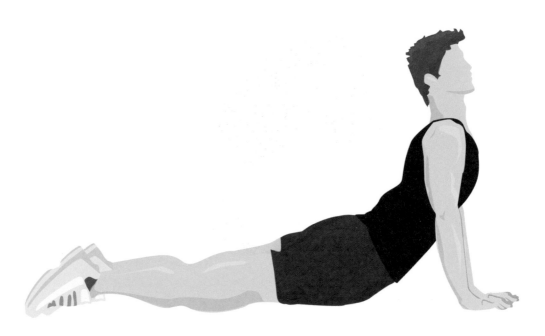

Instructions:

You might want to put a mat on the floor for this exercise. A yoga mat works well or a folded wool blanket.

Begin by lying on your belly, feet shoulder-width apart. Squeeze your buttock muscles together. Doing so will protect the lower spine and SI joint (sacro-iliac joint where the lower back meets the pelvis). Now plant both hands on the floor by your sides, about mid-rib height. Inhale, and on the next exhale roll your head and lift your chest off the mat. Breathe with ease. If your breath is not easy, back off the stretch.

You should feel a stretch in your abdominal region that may include the deep abdominal muscles crossing you're the front of your hips. Hold for about 15–20 seconds. Then release, resting completely on the mat for another half 15–20 seconds before moving again. This resting allows the newly stretched muscles to "re-set."

Safety:

If you feel any pinching in your shoulder or tingling in your hands or fingers, back off the stretch until these symptoms subside.

PYRAMID

Benefits:

Pyramid balances your hips and stretches your hamstrings and lower back.

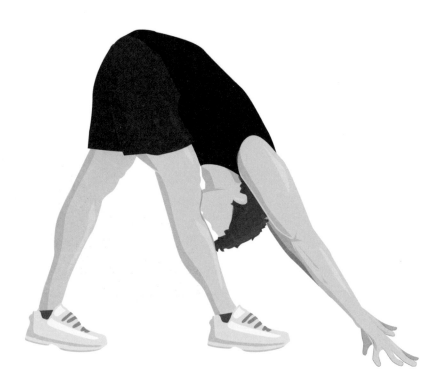

Instructions:

Begin with your right foot in front and your left foot behind, shoulder width apart with feet facing forwards. Stand tall and inhale. On an exhale, fold your body over your front foot by hinging at the hips, resting your hands gently on the front thigh. Keep your back straight, moving the chest toward the right knee. You will begin to feel a stretch in the hamstring muscles of the right (front) leg. Again, make sure to keep to the 60% rule.

If, in the beginning, the stretch is so intense that you can't keep your back straight, then try bending your right knee just a bit. Hold the stretch for about half a minute, breathing easily. You may find that the intensity of the stretch diminishes, and you can begin to straighten your right leg a bit.

After half a minute, on a next exhale, move back to an upright position. Switch legs and repeat on the other side.

Safety:

Do not do this exercise in sock feet or any leather soled shoe or slipper. Bare feet or good rubber-soled exercise shoes work best. A yoga mat will help your feet grip the floor.

KNEELING QUAD STRETCH

Benefits:

Kneeling quad stretch is a good stretch for the muscles in the front of your thighs and the hip flexors.

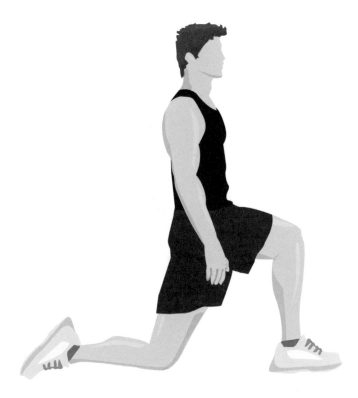

Instructions:

On a yoga mat, to protect your knees, kneel on your right knee with the top of the right foot lying on the floor. Place your left foot out in front of you so that your left thigh is parallel to the floor and your left knee is at a 90-degree angle. Now tuck your tail bone under like a "scared dog." In this position, lengthen the spine, as if there is a string pulling from the top of your head toward the ceiling—but your tailbone is still tucked.

Place your hands on your hips. On a next exhale, glide the pelvis forward to the hip flexors and front of thigh. When you feel a good (60%) stretch in the right hip and thigh, hold the stretch, breathing easily and gently, for about half a minute. As the stretch eases, you may be able to glide forward a bit more.

After about half a minute and on a next exhale, return to upright. Switch to the other side and repeat as above.

Safety:

To protect the low back, make sure to hold the tail bone tuck, keeping your spine long.

ARM OPENERS

Benefits:

Arm openers stretch your arms, chest, and shoulders

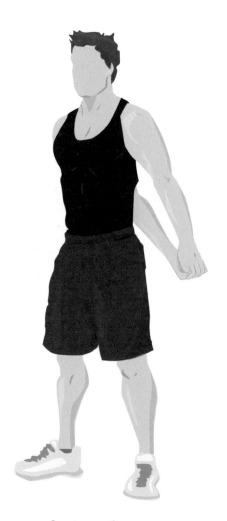

Instructions:

With your feet shoulder-width apart, interlace your fingers behind your tailbone with knuckles down. Stand tall with tail bone tucked and spine long. On an exhale, hinge forward at the hips to bend the chest toward the floor, while lifting the hands off the tail bone and up toward the ceiling. Open your chest toward the floor to expand the shoulder stretch. Hold for about half a minute. On a next exhale, lift back to standing position, bringing your hands to rest by your side.

Safety:

To protect your back during this exercise, make sure to keep your spine long and chest open toward the floor as you move into and out of the stretch, and as you hold the stretch.

If your hamstrings are too tight to stay in this stretch comfortably for half a minute, then bend your knees slightly.

WARM-UP STRETCHES
(10 MINUTES WITH DEEP BREATHING)

1. ARM OPENER
CHALLENGE 1 | *15 Seconds*
CHALLENGE 2 | *30 Seconds*
CHALLENGE 3 | *45 Seconds*

1. TRICEPS PULL
CHALLENGE 1 | *15 Seconds*
CHALLENGE 2 | *30 Seconds*
CHALLENGE 3 | *45 Seconds*

2. COBRA (ABDOMINAL STRETCH)
CHALLENGE 1 | *15 Seconds*
CHALLENGE 2 | *30 Seconds*
CHALLENGE 3 | *45 Seconds*

2. QUAD PULL
CHALLENGE 1 | *15 Seconds*
CHALLENGE 2 | *30 Seconds*
CHALLENGE 3 | *45 Seconds*

3. KNEELING QUAD STRETCH
CHALLENGE 1 | *15 Seconds*
CHALLENGE 2 | *30 Seconds*
CHALLENGE 3 | *45 Seconds*

3. PYRAMID
CHALLENGE 1 | *15 Seconds*
CHALLENGE 2 | *30 Seconds*
CHALLENGE 3 | *45 Seconds*

FULL BODY WORKOUT
(30 MINUTES WITH 10-30 SECOND REST)

1. ALTERNATING LUNGES
CHALLENGE 1 | *6 Repetitions x 3 Sets*
CHALLENGE 2 | *8 Repetitions x 3 Sets*
CHALLENGE 3 | *10 Repetitions x 3 Sets*

6. PULL UPS
CHALLENGE 1 | *4 Repetitions x 3 Sets*
CHALLENGE 2 | *8 Repetitions x 3 Sets*
CHALLENGE 3 | *12 Repetitions x 3 Sets*

2. SQUATS
CHALLENGE 1 | *6 Repetitions x 3 Sets*
CHALLENGE 2 | *8 Repetitions x 3 Sets*
CHALLENGE 3 | *10 Repetitions x 3 Sets*

7. DIPS
CHALLENGE 1 | *15 Repetitions x 3 Sets*
CHALLENGE 2 | *10 Repetitions x 3 Sets*
CHALLENGE 3 | *15 Repetitions x 3 Sets*

3. PUSH UPS
CHALLENGE 1 | *5 Repetitions x 3 Sets*
CHALLENGE 2 | *10 Repetitions x 3 Sets*
CHALLENGE 3 | *15 Repetitions x 3 Sets*

8. LEG LEVERS
CHALLENGE 1 | *5 Repetitions x 3 Sets*
CHALLENGE 2 | *10 Repetitions x 3 Sets*
CHALLENGE 3 | *15 Repetions x 3 Sets*

2. ARM HAULERS (SUPERMAN)
CHALLENGE 1 | *4 Repetitions x 3 Sets*
CHALLENGE 2 | *8 Repetitions x 3 Sets*
CHALLENGE 3 | *12 Repetitions x 3 Sets*

9. ABDOMINAL FLUTTER KICKS
CHALLENGE 1 | *5 Repetitions x 3 Sets*
CHALLENGE 2 | *10 Repetitions x 3 Sets*
CHALLENGE 3 | *15 Repetitions x 3 Sets*

3. PLANK
CHALLENGE 1 | *30 Seconds*
CHALLENGE 2 | *45 Seconds*
CHALLENGE 3 | *60 Seconds*

10. CALF RAISES
CHALLENGE 1 | *10 Repetitions x 3 Sets*
CHALLENGE 2 | *20 Repetitions x 3 Sets*
CHALLENGE 3 | *30 Repetitions x 3 Sets*

FROM LIFESTYLE CHANGES TO HEALTHY HABITS

We are creatures of habit. Difficulty with change seems to be a fact of human nature. My experience shows me unfortunately that only people who are seriously ill will make quick, decisive, and radical changes to diet and lifestyle because the extent of their illness is the one thing that will sufficiently motivate them. They do not want to die. A man who is just at the start of prostate disease—perhaps getting up only once during the night—typically finds it difficult to get motivated to make the changes necessary to keep the disease from getting worse or reversing it while he still can.

I encourage people to make slow, steady changes. Start what you know you can do. Get that first set of changes under your belt. Then take on another one that may seem more difficult.

If diet seems like a good first start to you, then go for it. But make the diet changes one step at a time. Don't do everything all at once. Start by cutting out dairy. Then cut out processed foods. Then sugar. Start adding more of the healthier components of my Prostate Specific diet. As each step feels rewarding, you will find it easier to take additional steps. You can add exercise later, and so on. The important thing is to make the changes and stay with them. Trying to bite off too many changes at once will inevitably result in backtracking to old ways.

For many people, the thought of making changes is actually far more daunting than actually doing it. You might think of habits as just a set of patterns we get into. Seen this way, you can start to think of drawing new patterns into your daily routine. These new patterns then start to become a more natural part of the fabric of your day-to-day life.

Provided that you really want to make these changes for your health, you will likely notice that the beginning effort gets progressively easier. So, let's say, for instance, that you have been in the habit of eating red meat every day and have never eaten vegetables really, other than potatoes—which are starches, not healthy veggies! You already gave up dairy and your favorite frozen pizza. Now it's time to make vegetables front and center on the plate and slide back on the amount of red meat. At first, you may think, "There's no way I can do this. I'll never enjoy eating again!"

But you forge ahead. You start with cutting red meat out 1 day a week, then two, and so on, until you are down to eating red meat only once per week. In the meantime, you are getting adventurous with veggies and salads. That first day without red meat may not be your favorite, but stay with it. Eventually, as you phase out the red meat to one day per week, you will notice that you actually enjoy the red meat more now because it's something to look forward to and no longer the mainstay of your meal. The same is true for adding vegetables. They may taste unfulfilling at first, but if you stay with it, soon you may find that you actually prefer vegetables over the red meat! This step-by-step re-patterning, plus a little willpower, perseverance, and perhaps a good dose of curiosity are all it takes to create a new habit over time.

Our experience with people who seriously undertake diet and lifestyle changes is that they feel improvements in their general well-being within a relatively short period. This improvement continues significantly over time. Studies support these experiences about new habits, and, importantly, they show also the impact that these changes have on prostate disease. The research strongly supports all the diet and lifestyle changes I have discussed thus far in this guide. I encourage you to take some time to peruse the extensive reference list for this guide, which will not only support your decision to make these changes. Reading these studies will help you also to become informed about your prostate and your health. And the more informed you are, the easier it is for you to discuss your care with your physician and make decisions that feel right for you.

DOING NOTHING IS NOT AN OPTION

Well, it is, of course, we always have choices. But if you have prostate disease of any kind, and you choose to you do nothing, the inconvenience, discomfort, and eventually pain will increase over the years. More importantly, your risk of the prostate disease escalating into cancer, and that cancer escalating to a point of becoming life-threatening will increase with every year that passes.

If you are in the early stages of prostate disease, don't wait to begin making the health-promoting changes that I have discussed. You may very well reverse the disease, and your health will be all the better for it. Many people experience the early stages of prostate disease as a wake-up call to take their health and their lives into their own hands. And often, these new habits are so life-changing that they wonder why they waited so long to take it upon themselves to make health priority #1.

PART 3:

A Simple Guide To Prostate Supplements

DIETARY SUPPLEMENTS AND LIFE CHANGES

I want to shift focus now to another mode of supporting prostate health: the use of dietary supplements. These include vitamins, minerals, healthy fats, probiotics, and phytonutrients (plant-based nutrients). Dietary supplements are sometimes referred to as "nutraceuticals" in contrast to pharmaceuticals, and there is a growing body of research supporting their efficacy in the treatment of chronic diseases. Our focus, of course, is on prostate disease and the promotion of your overall health on behalf of the health of your prostate. In the sections that follow, I detail a selection of dietary supplements that show promising results in clinical and lab studies. Increasingly, people are turning to nutraceuticals over pharmaceuticals to protection against chronic diseases, improvement of health, and for the many ways they support the body's natural functions.

Many drug companies and physicians will tell you that using dietary supplements to reverse disease is malarkey. And you may think so too, if you have been conditioned by conventional medicine to think that supplements provide anecdotal support at best and the only way to effectively manage disease is through pharmaceuticals and other more invasive or high-tech medical interventions. Drug companies and the medical establishment have worked together and persistently to make sure that we believe this line about "effective management."

Drug companies stand to gain by keeping us ensnared by a strong belief in their products and the fear that if we don't take them, we will get sicker and die. Why? It's simple. They profit financially.

With few exceptions, drug companies are in the business of managing disease, not curing it. This is so because of a flaw in approach, particularly when it comes to chronic diseases, such as prostate disease. Drugs target just one aspect of a disease, and conventional medicine is taught similarly do the same.

Some people refer to this strategy as the "broken part" model of medicine. I discussed this early on, using the car example. Something breaks. We take the car to the mechanic. The mechanic finds the broken part, presumably, fixes it, and we're on our way. Medicine, as it is practiced today, and drug companies, operate under this assumption. But this belief system does not tell the whole story.

I hope that by now in this guide I have given a good picture of how chronic disease develops and worsens. Prostate disease does not fit into a "broken part" model. A broken leg does, certainly. But prostate disease is chronic and a long time in the making. To cure prostate disease, as I have emphasized a number of times, we need to go to the source. And, at least for now, research is telling us increasingly that inflammation and hormone imbalance are places to look. But even that is too simple! Already, pharmaceuticals target inflammation and hormone imbalances.

We need to take a long look at why systemic inflammation and hormone balances are happening and how they are interconnected. If we think of the body as an ecosystem where everything is connected, then it is not difficult to see that systemic inflammation and hormone imbalances are not two separate things going on in the body. They are linked processes of the greater "whole."

Dietary supplements work in sync the body to restore the whole, instead of just targeting separate broken parts. They synergize with the body's natural processes. If you think about it, this synergy between our bodies and natural supplements makes sense. We humans grew out of nature after all.

Yet, with depleted soil, even organic produce and pasture-raised animals are lacking in the quantity of "micro-nutrients" that are essential for a healthy immune system. By micro-nutrients, I am referring to essential vitamins, trace minerals, fatty acids, probiotics, and phytonutrients—ingredients found in dietary supplements. When Hippocrates insisted, "Let food be thy medicine and medicine by thy food," he was living during a time when people relied on a much wider variety of foods than we eat today, including many plants no longer found in our diets. It was not unusual for people to make teas and other concentrated plant-based concoctions as a part of a health regimen. If we think about supplements in this way, then we can imagine them boosting the variety of foods that we ingest.

A point I want to make is this: when thinking about supplementing our health regimen with dietary supplements, we can't rely on how we have been taught to think about over-the-counter (OTC) and prescription drugs. The "target the broken part" approach won't do here. Supplements are not "fix-it" pills that give us permission to keep eating junk and being sedentary and stressed. They must be part of a coordinated effort that includes changes in diet and lifestyle. It is wholly unrealistic to continue all the same habits that, over decades, have caused disease and simply pop a handful of supplements in your mouth every day imagining that you will suddenly be free of the disease and its symptoms. This "keep doing what you're doing" approach may be fine for pharmaceuticals, but no one ever said they would cure your prostate disease. In fact, the benefits from dietary supplements can be partly and even wholly counteracted by continuing disease-forming habits.

Supplements are not magic bullets that suddenly and miraculously will cure prostate disease. Pharmaceutical companies can give us these expectations because drugs sometimes do remove symptoms almost immediately. Supplements, on the other hand, may take some time because they work in tandem with the body's natural healing processes. It took a long time for prostate disease to develop. It may take some time for supplements, in conjunction with diet, exercise, and lifestyle changes, to undo the deteriorating effects of these disease processes. Making these dietary and lifestyle changes restore us to the body's natural way.

What I am emphasizing is the importance of making health priority #1. Supplements are one aspect of this health regimen, but they do not make right our bad habits!

Research on Dietary Supplements

There is an image in the public mind that pharmaceutical drugs are derived from very serious and reliable research while dietary supplements are preparations that come from unscientific folklore. But this perspective is completely biased and serves only the pharmaceutical industry and any provider in the medical establishment who receives some benefit from big drug companies, whether that's through meals, paid travel to conferences, or even funding for research on pharmaceuticals. It is true that there is a heavy regulation by the FDA on the testing of pharmaceuticals. Strange as it may sound, big pharmaceutical corporations benefit from this tight regulation. It creates a large financial barrier that keeps the competition at bay, justifies their demand for a monopoly protected by patents and further regulation, and enables them to profit at obscene levels. Unfortunately, drug science is also subverted by corporate funding that pays for the overwhelming majority of research. So, what we have is a biased system from the start that makes every effort to keep it that way.

Yet, the ancient use of plants and foods for healing has captured the attention of the mainstream who is reaching increasingly for a natural approach to their health issues. As a result, a great deal of modern scientific investigation is now actively researching the use of nutraceuticals as medicine. Huge pharmaceutical corporations have no stake in this research. Much of it is independently funded, conducted with strict scientific rigor by highly trained scientists and increasingly, medical researchers. While the field of medicine has been painfully slow to open up to the benefits of nutraceuticals, the interest by the public is pushing medical research in this direction. There are far fewer of these studies and sturdy roadblocks erected by the pharmaceutical corporations who stand to lose—because they can't get a patent on a plant! And, as I have iterated many times in this guide, physicians are painfully slow to come around for all the reasons I discussed in Part I about the old establishment, reputations, and profit.

What you will find in the sections that follow regarding the use of dietary supplements for treating prostate disease is backed by solid laboratory and clinical research that is rigorous and ongoing not only in the field but also by me and my team at Ben's Natural Health. Each of the ingredients in the dietary supplements listed below have been thoroughly researched for efficacy. While many researchers are still trying to figure out how many of these phytonutrients work and are encouraging this physiological research, there are scores of studies with large sample sizes that show that they do. These studies inform the formulations of the dietary supplements that I describe below. For readers who may be interested in reading more about the research on dietary supplements, there are many references in the bibliography at the end of this text that will surely be of interest to you. For others who may not be as interested in reading these studies or abstracts to them, I encourage you to look at the bibliography if for no other reason than to see how extensive it is.

Discerning Supplement Quality

There are hosts of vitamin and mineral formulas on the market. Because it can be difficult to discern the quality of these products, most people rely on brand name, or they buy at what they believe to be a reasonable price level. It is important to remember that lower cost products may skimp on dosage, and this lower dosage equates with lower quality and lesser support for the body's tissues and healthy functioning.

I get e-mails most days from men who read the earlier edition of this guide and purchased supplements based on the nutrients that I recommend. They complain that the supplements have not worked for them. The fact is that there is more to a nutrient than the name. What these men seem to have in common is that they bought the cheapest supplement they could find containing the nutrient that I recommend. I understand the impulse. But not all supplements are equal even if the name is the same.

My supplements work for most men because I do not cut any corners. Plain and simple. I use only the finest quality ingredients and standardize dosages based on the studies that have shown these nutrients to work. If these practices make my supplements a bit more expensive than some of my competition who do cut corners, well, I have to say, that is fine with me.

Permit me to give you a few examples that speak to quality. Labels can be very misleading. It is perfectly legitimate to label Alpha D Tocopherol as vitamin E, but this ingredient is the synthetic version of vitamin E, and synthetic is useless. Only mixed natural tocopherols as vitamin E are actually beneficial to the body, and they happen to be more expensive, not only for the consumer, but also for us to purchase. Now how is the average Joe supposed to know that?

Next, there are plenty of supplements on the market that mention an ingredient, but the ingredient is not in the bottle. Then there is the problem that most labels do not tell you the source of an extract or its level of concentration, so you can have two supplements, one at 10% extract and another at 90% extract, but the label will be exactly the same. With Ben's Total Health for the Prostate, for example, you get 750mg of 90% extract Beta-Sitosterol, and my label actually specifies that. The same is true for the vitamin E in this supplement. You will see in the list of ingredients I provide below that my Ben's Total Health for the Prostate uses only mixed natural tocopherols even though they are far more expensive to source than synthetic vitamin E. And many multivitamin supplements say on the label 'vitamin D'. But the vitamin D that you need is vitamin D3. How many ordinary shoppers would know the difference? If the label does not say vitamin D3, then this particular vitamin D supplement will do you no good.

One final example on this point: I wonder if most people know how many different trace minerals they should be taking or that chelated minerals are those that have been processed with amino acids, which makes them more bioavailable. Chelated minerals make it possible to actually benefit from them. They are more expensive, though, which is why most multi-mineral supplements do not contain chelated minerals. The minerals in Ben's supplements are all chelated, to be optimally beneficial. I could go on, but I think I have made my point. It is important to buy from a trusted source. Ask questions. Become an informed consumer.

My factory in Seattle uses the highest standard of GMP (good manufacturing practices) for quality control. So, we do a pre-production laboratory analysis of every ingredient before it is added to a supplement. Plus, there is a follow-up analysis after production to check again that everything on the label is 100% accurate. I can guarantee that whatever my label states is an accurate representation of the contents of my supplement.

Ben's dietary supplements are extracted from the highest quality, natural ingredients and freshly harvested herbs, using the most stringent, cold-pressed extraction methods to optimize each supplement for dosage and "bioavailability." Bioavailability refers to the extent to which the supplement makes its way into the body's tissues rather than being flushed out as waste from the intestinal tract. Minerals are chelated with amino acids, and none of the vitamins in our formulations are synthetic. Our preparations maximize the potency and efficacy of each supplement. For these reasons, I believe our products are the best on the market.

What is important, of course, is to experience for yourself what these supplements do for you. If you are confused about any of the options or information I provide here, please feel free to email us at any time. If you do reach out to us with a question, make sure to give us as much information as possible about your condition. We are always happy to assist.

In what follows, I detail all the information you need to know about Ben's supplements. Considerable research has gone into each of them and their potential benefits. Part of the reason I provide so much detail is to be completely transparent so you know what you're getting and why.

As a result, you will find quite a bit of information below. Some of you reading this guide will be interested in all that information. Others will prefer to get the gist and move on. I organized this chapter for both readers in mind. First, I provide you detailed information about Beta-Sitosterol, which I believe is the most powerful plant nutrient for prostate health. Beta-Sitosterol is incorporated into several of my supplements, as you will see. Then, I provide a "go-to" list of Ben's supplements that I personally recommend in order of priority. I provide a summary about how each supplement can help and then offer more details for those of you who want to know more. For the "just the gist" reader, you may want to simply read the summary for each product. I also provide a list of nutrients that I personally believe are not so helpful but have received a lot of attention as dietary supplements for prostate disease.

In the interest of full disclosure, the supplement formulations that I recommend are preparations I formulated myself and that I sell at www.bensnaturalhealth.com. I started formulating these supplements because when I was diagnosed with prostate disease, there was nothing on the market that was of the quality I knew I needed to solve my prostate issues. I wanted to lower my PSA, shrink my prostate, get back to sleeping full nights, and enjoy my health once again. I knew that to achieve these results naturally, I needed the best quality food supplements.

I never intended to sell these supplements. I was already retired. I always intended them to be just for me. That's why I didn't cut any corners or skimp on dose size or ingredient quality. It turns out that these preparations I made for myself became the best quality supplements and ended up becoming sellable products. Over the last twenty years, my clinical nutrition team and I have improved, enhanced, and reformulated the supplements to make them even better, but at their core, these are still the same supplements that cured my own prostate disease. And they are the ones that have been used by hundreds of thousands of men to restore their own health.

Beta-Sitosterol: The Most Important Supplement for Prostate Health

Clinical research has shown that the most powerful, clinically proven, and effective nutritional supplement for prostate health is a common plant sterol called Beta-Sitosterol. Sterols are steroid alcohols that are naturally occurring in all plants, animals, and fungi, as well as some bacteria. Literally every vegetable you eat contains Beta-Sitosterol. It serves a vital role in the structure of each cell's membrane and in the signalling pathways into, out of, and between cells. Cholesterol is the most common type of sterol in animals.

Recent research has looked at Beta-Sitosterol's role in supporting numerous issues associated with prostate disease. Numbers of studies have shown Beta-Sitosterol to be effective in reducing urinary urgency, frequency and night-time waking, as well as improving starting and stopping and strengthening urinary flow. Studies have also shown that Beta-Sitosterol binds with estrogen receptors. As we know from the earlier discussion on estrogen, too much it can off-set the hormone balance and contribute to growth of the prostate.

Other studies point to Beta-Sitosterol's role in reducing boosting the immune system and reducing inflammation. As with hormone imbalance, we have already discussed the role that chronic systemic inflammation plays in prostate disease, including prostate cancer, which brings me to my next point about this potent phytonutrient. Studies also show that Beta-Sitosterol may interfere with many of the signalling pathways in cancer cells, including cell proliferation and metastasis, and may even act on the pathways that signal the cancer cell to die.

The difficulty with Beta-Sitosterols has to do with getting enough and in combination with the right amount of fatty acids. The problem is that the Beta-Sitosterol compounds are expensive, much more expensive than the fatty acids. As a result, there are many products on the market that are upwards of 70% fatty acids, with less than 30% Beta-Sitosterols. These products are ineffective and won't help you with prostate disease. Don't waste your money on lesser products.

For Beta-Sitosterol to be effective, it needs to be at a ratio of 90% plant sterols to 10% fatty acids. Without the fatty acids, these plant nutrients become unstable and are useless, but only about 10% is necessary to stabilize the supplement. Always check the ingredient label, and if the product does not disclose the ratio on the label, you should assume it's a cheap blend that won't help you. When it comes to your health, it's always worth spending a little more and getting an effective supplement.

I have included Beta-Sitosterol in several of my products, including Ben's Total Health and Ben's

Total Health Advanced for the Prostate. While Beta-Sitosterol is powerful, it cannot restore your health on its own. No single nutrient can do that. So, I have included other ingredients, which have been studied extensively, in these two supplements, and I recommend other supplements that I include in this list, which I would prioritize as follows:

1. Ben's Total Health for the Prostate OR Ben's Total Health Advanced for the Prostate
2. Ben's Prostate Healer Tincture
3. Ben's Prostate Power
4. Ben's Prostate Health Program
5. Ben's Male Boost Tincture
6. Ben's Estro Clear
7. Rejuvenayte Plus

PROSTATE SUPPLEMENTS

It is not uncommon for some men to end up on my website, or reading one of my articles, or even reading this exact page of my book, without really knowing what is wrong with their prostate. Sometimes they know a little, sometimes they know nothing at all. Sometimes all they know is that they are waking up during the night. Other times their doctor may have mentioned that their prostate is enlarged during their last health check-up. Either way, my team and I often speak to men who don't really know what is wrong with their prostate or why their health has deteriorated. If you find yourself in a similar situation, then hopefully this book has already provided you with a great deal of information about the origins and causes of your prostate disease.

My team and I have spent two decades talking to men and helping them with their prostate. And what we have noticed is that men who have been diagnosed with prostate disease have more questions about their health, not less. You might think that their doctors would have answered all their questions when they were diagnosed. However, the reality is that doctors are often so busy, so swamped with patients, that they only have time to throw a few pills at you. This can lead to people taking multiple medications everyday, with only the vaguest notion of what they are for. More often than not, men simply know that their prostate is enlarged, or that they have a high PSA. Sometimes they know their PSA level, other times they don't. And even if they know their PSA level, they often don't know what it means.

This uncertainty about the exact nature of their prostate disease often results in them feeling trapped. Unsure of what the problem is, they don't feel confident about questioning their medication, shopping for supplements or changing their diet and lifestyle. Because they don't understand what is wrong with them, they cannot act to fix it.

Because of this, my clinical nutrition team has put together an Online Personalized Prostate Health Assessment that you can find on our website. It takes 5-8 minutes to complete and asks only a few basic prostate, health and lifestyle questions. After completing it you will get a complete 3 page report that can be used to help you or your doctor make informed decisions about your prostate health and your treatment plan.

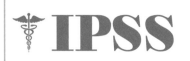 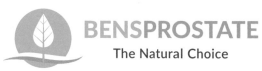 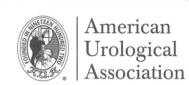

THE PROSTATE HEALTH ASSESSMENT

The assessment was developed using the International Prostate Symptom Score and is an enhanced version of the assessment used by the American Urological Association. Our Prostate Health Assessment is the result of a year long collaboration between ourselves and several doctors, nutritionists, and prostate health experts.

Taking 5 minutes to complete the assessment will give you an in-depth, personalized report that will tell you exactly how healthy your prostate is - and exactly the steps you can take to ensure a happy, healthy, disease-free future surrounded by your loved ones.

WHAT IS IN THE PROSTATE HEALTH ASSESSMENT ?

You will receive a wide range of important prostate health indicators as part of the assessment, along with practical advice and personalized dietary recommendations. The report will be delivered digitally straight to your inbox within minutes of completing it. Your reports are kept confidential, in line with American and European data laws. You can choose to download your report as a PDF or access it online with a unique PIN that will be emailed to you. This allows you to take multiple assessments over the course of your treatments and to track the real time improvements in your prostate health.

The assessment explains what your PSA score really means and how it relates to other men your age and in your risk bracket. Using the assessment, you can discover whether or not you are at a higher risk of developing prostate cancer...without having to leave your chair!

The assessment also generates a Urinary Symptom Score which helps you understand how severe your symptoms are. In addition you will receive personalized recommendations on how you can reduce or alleviate them.

The assessment also calculates Body Mass Index Score (BMI) and explains the degree to which they may or may not be affecting your prostate health. It will also provide you with diet and lifestyle advice, and if you need it, you can get further personalized advice from our specialized team of nutritionists for free.

Finally, the assessment addresses your main prostate health concerns in order to provide you with the information you need to make informed decisions about your health and treatment plan.

If you'd like to get a personalized prostate health assessment today, it take only a few minutes, costs nothing and is a valuable tool for you or your doctor. Just visit: www.bensprostate.com/e/prostate-health-assessment

Ben's Total Health for the Prostate is the most important single supplement I recommend to any man over fifty, not only men with active prostate disease. If you are in early stages of prostate disease and your doctor is sounding warning signals that your PSA levels are on the rise, then there is no more comprehensive supplement on the market to address all the factors that might be working in tandem to cause deterioration of your prostate gland. If you have prostate cancer, this supplement will not lower your PSA, but, if your cancer is localized to the prostate, and has not penetrated the outer wall of the gland; then Ben's Total Health for the Prostate may be beneficial in reducing the chances of the cancer progressing.

PROSTATE SUPPLEMENTS

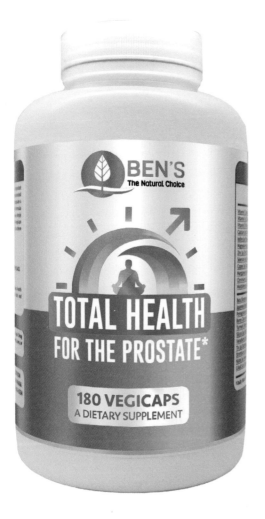

	Ingredients	% Daily Value	Amount Per Serving
	SUPPLEMENT FACTS (SERVING SIZE 6 VEGICAPS)		
5	Vitamin C	100%	60mg
2	Vitamin D3	1250%	5000IU
14	Vitamin E-Mixed Tocopherals	1333%	400IU
7	Calcium Chelate	5%	50mg
22	Iodine Chelate	100%	150mcg
15	Magnesium Chelate	18%	70mg
8	Zinc Chelate	100%	15mg
9	Selenium Chelate	100%	70mg
10	Copper Chelate	100%	2mg
12	Manganese Chelate	100%	2mg
21	Chromium Picolinate	11%	13mcg
11	Molybdenum Chelate	100%	75mcg
1	Beta Sitosterol (90%)	N/A	750mcg
13	Quercertin (95%)	N/A	200mg
3	Ellagic Acid (40%)	N/A	200mg
4	Boron Citrate	N/A	150mg
6	Turmeric 4:1	N/A	62.5mg
17	Silicon Chelate	N/A	10mg
16	Vanadium Chelate	N/A	1mg
18	Tin Chelate	N/A	100mcg
20	Strontium Chelate	N/A	100mcg
23	Nickel Chelate	N/A	100mcg
19	Cobalt Chelate	N/A	10mcg

SUMMARY:

Ben's Total Health for the Prostate is a full-spectrum multi-mineral complex with clinically proven anti-inflammatory, antioxidant, and anti-cancer nutrients from 100% natural ingredients. Ben's Total Health for the Prostate is formulated with natural 5-alpha-reductase inhibitors and powerful ingredients to lower DHT levels and reduce the size of the prostate gland. This formulation works synergistically to get at the inflammatory and hormone imbalances contributing to prostate disease. This multi-faceted approach to prostate disease helps to reduce night-time waking, urinary symptoms, improve urinary flow and speed, and ensure overall health of prostate, bladder, and kidneys.

ACTIVE INGREDIENTS:

1 **Beta-Sitosterol (90% Sterols):** Improves urinary symptoms and acts as a natural inhibitor of 5 alpha-reductase enzyme to reduce prostate size.

2 **Vitamin D3 (Cholecalciferol):** May decrease the risk of developing prostate cancer by killing cancer cells and preventing them from spreading.

3 **Pomegranate (Ellagic acid):** Pomegranate is high in ellagic acid, a natural anti-cancer agent.

4 **Boron Glycine Complex:** An important trace mineral, boron improves the body's use of estrogen, testosterone, and vitamin D, and thereby, importantly restoring male to female hormone balance. It also reduces inflammation, supports the immune system, boosts absorption of magnesium, and may have anti-carcinogenic properties.

5 **Vitamin C:** Repairs tissues throughout the body, protects against infections, age-related conditions, and may lower the risk of prostate cancer.

6 **Turmeric Root (Curcumin):** Curcumin is a strong natural anti-inflammatory. It also combats prostate and bladder infections, reduces prostate size, and may inhibit the development of cancer cells.

7 **Calcium:** The most abundant mineral in the body, calcium is needed by every cell in order to function optimally. Promotes optimal heart and bone health, muscle function, nerve transmission, and importantly for the prostate, hormone secretion.

8 **Zinc:** The most abundant mineral in the prostate, zinc is vital for maintaining prostate health and combatting BPH and prostate cancer. Insufficient levels of zinc negatively impact the immune system.

9 **Selenium:** An important trace mineral, selenium is a natural immune booster that may lower chances of developing prostate cancer or the worsening and spread of it. In fact, studies link low selenium intake with prostate cancer.

10 **Copper:** An essential trace mineral, is a powerful antioxidant, fighting free radical DNA damage while boosting the immune system. A healthy immune system is crucial for a healthy prostate. Copper also helps provide energy to cells—which translates to energy levels for you! Lastly, copper helps to maintain nerve health.

11 **Molybdenum:** Helps repair and maintain vital bodily processes by breaking down certain substances, including proteins, such as PSA. Your body can store molybdenum for only a limited time for future use, so regular consumption is critical. Although molybdenum is known to be necessary for health, recently it has come to the attention of medical researchers for use as a treatment for a large number of medical conditions. These studies are preliminary but point to the importance of molybdenum.

12 **Manganese:** A key trace mineral, manganese is involved in countless functions of the body, including the immune system. It supports production of sperm and sex hormones, boosting libido, and maintaining prostate and sexual health. Also supports everyday brain function. An estimated 40% of Americans do not consume sufficient levels of manganese in their diets.

13 **Japanese Sophora Flower Buds (Quercetin):** A natural antioxidant that has been shown to relieve symptoms of prostatitis and BPH while also promoting cellular health in general.

14 **Vitamin E-mixed Tocopherols:** A powerful, fat-soluble antioxidant, vitamin E is essential for a healthy prostate and may reduce the risk of cancer, but more studies are needed to confirm this possible benefit. What the evidence does clearly support, however, is that when taken as a well-formulated and balanced supplement, vitamin E is essential to health.

15 **Magnesium:** Required for more than 300 biochemical reactions in the body, magnesium increases the bioavailability of testosterone produced by the body while also improving nerve function. A natural muscle relaxant, magnesium is also helpful for restful sleep.

16 **Vanadium:** A "micro-mineral," meaning your body only needs a minuscule amount, vanadium may inhibit and/or slow the proliferation of prostate cancer cells. It has other health-promoting properties as well, including being "insulin-mimetic," meaning it mimics insulin, which may make it an important mineral for treatment of metabolic disorders and diabetes.

17 **Silicon:** Another trace mineral, silicon is essential for building healthy tissues. It also promotes whole-body health and reduces the risk of heart disease, strokes, and Alzheimer's.

18 **Tin (Stannous Chloride):** Reduces fatigue, improves energy, well-being and mood, and promotes full nights' sleep.

19 **Cobalt:** Plays an important role in the production of coenzymes that are vital to prostate and bodily health. Cobalt also maintains nerve and red blood cell health.

20 **Strontium:** Works alongside calcium. It also is instrumental, therefore, in preventing bone loss

and reducing the risk of osteoporosis.

Chromium: Normalizes blood sugar levels, which is important for prostate health, because high levels of sugar promote inflammation, and in the case of prostate cancer, high levels of sugar mean ready "food" for cancer cells. Chromium also increases fat metabolism, helping to maintain optimal weight, and as an added bonus, it may improve cognitive function by improving insulin activity in the brain.

Iodine: Promotes healthy thyroid function and metabolism while also reducing the symptoms of aging. Research is investigating the role of iodine deficiency in cancer risk.

Nickel: Necessary for absorbing iron and maintaining blood and bone health.

PROVEN RESULTS OR 100% OF YOUR MONEY BACK!

I believe that Total Health for The Prostate can help everyone improve their symptoms, shrink their prostate and improve their health. Which is why I give the strongest money back guarantee in the industry.

It's a simple, iron clad guarantee. Get a PSA test, try "Total Health for the Prostate" for 90 days, get another PSA test… If your PSA levels and prostate health have not improved we will return 100% of your money.

No other supplement manufacturer in the world gives an ironclad laboratory backed guarantee.

* In cases of cancer or surgical damage to the prostate I cannot guarantee that Total Health will lower your PSA. If any of the below conditions are met, or the testing requirements are not met, the guarantee is voided.

1. You have been diagnosed with prostate cancer
2. You are currently taking prescription medication for prostate cancer
3. You have had a prostatectomy
4. You have had surgery on your urethra, prostate or bladder
5. You last PSA test showed a result higher than 8

* The Before and After PSA tests must be taken no earlier than 30 days before starting Total Health and no more than 30 days after stopping taking Total Health or it will not be accepted for the purpose of claiming the 100% money back guarantee.

Ben's Total Health Advanced for the Prostate contains all the ingredients in Ben's Total Health with the same high quality of ingredients and dosage. In addition, Ben's Total Health Advanced is clinically formulated to protect DNA and fight oxidative damage. This supplement helps lower the risk of prostate cancer and prevents cell mutation and tumor growth.

PROSTATE SUPPLEMENTS

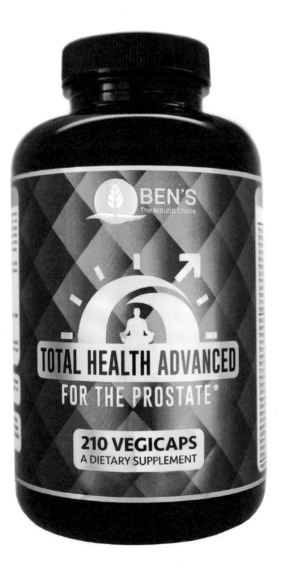

SUPPLEMENT FACTS (SERVING SIZE 6 VEGICAPS)

Ingredients	% Daily Value	Amount Per Serving
Vitamin C	100%	60mg
Vitamin D3	1250%	5000IU
Vitamin E-Mixed Tocopherals	1333%	400IU
Calcium Chelate	5%	50mg
Iodine Chelate	100%	150mcg
Magnesium Chelate	18%	70mg
Zinc Chelate	100%	15mg
Selenium Chelate	100%	70mg
Copper Chelate	100%	2mg
Manganese Chelate	100%	2mg
Chromium Picolinate	11%	13mcg
Molybdenum Chelate	100%	75mcg
Beta Sitosterol (90%)	N/A	750mcg
Quercertin (95%)	N/A	200mg
Ellagic Acid (40%)	N/A	200mg
Turmeric 4:1	N/A	150mg
Silicon	N/A	62.5mg
Vanadium	N/A	10mg
Boron Glycine Complex	N/A	1mg
Tin	N/A	100mcg
Nickel	N/A	100mcg
Strontium	N/A	100mcg
Cobalt	N/A	10mcg
Pygeum (Bark)	N/A	150mg
Ginger (Root)	N/A	80mg
Rosemary (Leaf)	N/A	75mg
Holy Basil (Leaf)	N/A	50mg
Japanase Fleeceflower (Root)	N/A	40mg
Chinese Goldthread (Root)	N/A	20mg
Barberry (Root)	N/A	20mg
Oregano (Leaf)	N/A	20mg
Chinese Skullcap (Root)	N/A	100mg

ACTIVE INGREDIENTS:

In addition to all the ingredients in Ben's Total Health for the Prostate, this premium prostate supplement contains:

Rosemary Leaf (Rosmarinic Acid): Improves urinary symptoms and fights BPH. May promote prostate cell cancer death.

Barbary Root (Berberine): Has been shown to inhibit prostate cancer cell proliferation. **Goldthread Chinese:** Works synergistically with turmeric (curcumin) to inhibit prostate cancer cell proliferation.

Holy Basil Leaf (Ursolic Acid): Simultaneously targets multiple signaling pathways to suppress proliferation and induce cancer cell death. Holy basil (Ocimum sanctum) has also been shown to have anti-stress effects, as well as anti-inflammatory and anti-microbial properties.

Oregano Leaf: Extremely potent anti-cancer agent. In studies, oregano oil extracts have shown to have strong inhibitory effects on existing cancer cell viability.

Chinese Skull Cap (Baicalin): Immune booster that may inhibit cancer cell proliferation and induces cancer cell death.

Pygeum Africanum: Improves urinary symptoms and fights BPH. May promote prostate cancer cell death.

Japanese Fleece Flower (Reservatrol): You may recall from Part 2's discussion on Salvestrols that they are activated by cancer cells and in turn, produce byproducts that are toxic to cancer cells, which destroys them. Reservatrol is one of the most powerful Salvestrols.

A FEW ADDITIONAL NOTES ABOUT BEN'S TOTAL HEALTH AND BEN'S TOTAL HEALTH ADVANCED FOR THE PROSTATE:

Both these supplements contain vitamin E in the form of natural, mixed tocopherols, which is the most effective form of vitamin E supplementation. Research has suggested that mixed tocopherols, in conjunction with selenium, may reduce the risk of contracting prostate cancer. Hence, these supplements also contain selenium. Synthetic vitamin E pales in comparison on efficacy. Similarly, typical mineral formulations contain only a handful of the most common minerals. It is important to have the full range of minerals, as is found in this formulation. Also, these supplements use only the chelated form of minerals, which makes them more bioavailable, if a bit costlier. But if the minerals are not absorbed into the body (i.e., they are not bioavailable), then they are worthless.

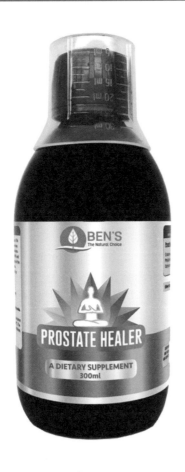

SUPPLEMENT FACTS

Serving Size: 10ML | Servings Per Container: 30

Proprietary Ayurvedic Herbal Blend:

Crataeva, Asparagus, Bauhinia, Curcuma Longa, Phyllanthus Embelica, Tribulus, Boerhaavia Difusa, Ocimum Sanctum, Withania Somifera.

PROSTATE SUPPLEMENTS

SUMMARY:

Ben's Prostate Healer Tincture is a scientifically refined Ayurvedic herbal prostate complex, a proprietary blend of 9 potent phytonutrients that goes to work directly on the entire male reproductive system and genitalia positively impacting prostate health by supporting the immune system and balancing hormonal levels.

Tinctures are a concentrated form of herbs extracted in an alcohol base. The herbs in Ben's Prostate Healer Tincture are cold pressed and macerated and preserved in pharmaceutical grade alcohol for optimal quality and standardization of dosing. The extraction process concentrates the active phytonutrients from the plant, producing six-times the effectiveness and bioavailability of the herbs as they occur naturally and would be consumed otherwise.

The beauty of tinctures is that they can be absorbed sublingually (under the tongue), bypassing the gastrointestinal system. This is particularly helpful for people who have "malabsorption" problems, meaning the lining of the gut is compromised, and nutrients are often lost in the process of digestion.

Sublingual administration of tinctures means that many of the nutrients enter the bloodstream immediately and are delivered more quickly and effectively throughout the body—even for people who do not have absorption problems. As an aside, if you have been existing on standard American fare, however, you can probably anticipate that your gut lining is damaged and that you have some level of compromised absorption.

Ben's Prostate Healer Tincture is formulated to re-establish a healthy estrogen–testosterone balance by supplying phytoestrogen compounds that mimic the action of estrogen, which, as we know plays an important role in causing BPH. Phytoestrogens compete with natural estrogens on the estrogen receptors of cells. By binding to these receptors, phytoestrogens prevent the negative impact on your prostate of estrogen circulating in the bloodstream. Phytoestrogens also discourage excessive estrogen production. Ben's Prostate Healer Tincture also inhibits an enzyme that converts testosterone to DHT (dihydrotestosterone), which, as you will recall from Part 1, binds to receptors in prostate cells and stimulates tissue growth. This growth constricts the urethra and leads to urinary disturbances. When Ben's Prostate Healer Tincture blocks the production of DHT, it prevents prostate growth.

Ben's Prostate Healer Tincture also provides nutrients that inhibit protein deposits, which obstruct prostate ducts and reduce prostate function. With the extract of Varuna, a classic bladder tonic, this tincture also purges the urinary tract, which boosts kidney efficiency, tones bladder tissue, and decreases residual urine volume. As such, it may also improve the symptoms related to prostatitis. Ben's Prostate Healer Tincture enhances the immune system. It does so by removing toxins from your blood, regulating the production of polyamine and prostaglandins (powerful immune-suppressants produced in the prostate), curtailing inflammation, elevating mast cell (special immune cells) levels, and thwarting cell proliferation. As such, Ben's Prostate Healer Tincture may serve as a potential agent in reducing cancer risk.

Ben's Prostate Healer Tincture is the safest and most effective means for you to experience a total rejuvenation of your prostate health. It works very effectively in conjunction with my Ben's Total Health or Ben's Total Health Advanced. These formulations are synergistic—meaning they work together in a manner in which "the sum is greater than the parts."

ACTIVE INGREDIENTS:

Because Ben's Prostate Healer Tincture is a blend of herbal concentrates from Ayurvedic science, backed by clinical studies, I list the Sanskrit name first followed by the English translation for each of the 9 ingredients.

Shatavari (Asparagus racemosus): A rejuvenating herb that soothes and nurtures the reproductive system and helps to reduce inflammation, which helps to reduce problems with urinary flow. It contains saponins, Shatavarin I to IV, phytoestrogen compounds. As I have discussed, phytoestrogens compete with natural estrogen at the estrogen receptor sites, reducing the potential for it to contribute to prostate growth and enlargement. Research indicates that Shatavari inhibits protein deposits in the lumen of the prostate. Long-term accumulation of proteins obstructs the prostate ducts. Other positive effects of Shatavari include detoxifying the blood by supporting liver function and metabolic processes.

Punarnava (Boerhavia diffusa): Contains Beta-Sitosterol and Ursolic acid, as well as vitamins D and E (all are ingredients the importance of which I discussed above). Research indicates Punarnava helps regulate the production of polyamine and prostaglandins, which are powerful immuno-suppressants that are produced in the prostate. Ursolic acid has anti-inflammatory properties and may reduce inflammation of the prostate and urethra. And you will recall that Beta-Sitosterol helps also to support and balance the healthy flow of urine. Throughout India, Punarnava is also used to stimulate liver function and promote healthy blood circulation, giving it added whole-health benefits.

Kanchanara (Bauhinia variegata): Kanchanara is used widely in Ayurvedic medicine for supporting the healthy functioning of the prostate gland. Kanchanara has a two-fold effect on DHT. First, it inhibits 5-alpha-reductase, which converts testosterone to DHT, so it, in effect, helps to reduce the amount of DHT. Second, it blocks whatever amount DHT is there from binding to prostate cells, thereby preventing prostate enlargement and the constriction of the urethra that can follow. In this way, Kanchanara supports healthy urine flow.

Gokshura (Tribulus terrestri): Gokshura contains a plethora of vitamins, minerals, and phytonutrients, including Beta-Sitosterol. Gokshura stimulates the production of the Luteinizing Hormone (LH). When LH levels are elevated, the natural production of testosterone also increases— by more than 50% in some cases, after 30 days of Gokshura administration. By promoting the production of the testosterone, Gokshura works with the body's natural equilibrium to help men achieve their strength and muscular potential, as well as libido and virility. Research indicates Gokshura can significantly improve the quantity and quality of sperm. Traditionally, it has also been used to ease painful, burning sensations during urination. Added health benefits include a stimulating effect on the liver, helping to convert cholesterol and fats into hormones and energy.

Varuna (Crateva nurvala): Ancient Ayurvedic practitioners used Varuna as an internal purifier that helped maintain homeostasis and balance. Varuna has been the herb of choice for maintaining healthy a urinary tract and bladder function. A bladder tonic that purges the urinary tract and improves kidney efficiency, Varuna helps to rid urine from the body more efficiently. It also helps prevent the formation of stones in the urinary tract.

Tulasi (Ocimum tenuiflorum): Like Gokushura, Tulasi is rich in an array of vitamins, minerals, and potent phytonutrients, including vitamin C, Beta-carotene, calcium, phosphoric acid, and Beta-Sitosterol. Often referred to as an adaptogen, these components work synergistically to support the body's natural physiology as a whole. Tulasi is frequently used in Ayurvedic medicine to treat common ailments, because it has antibacterial, antifungal, and antiviral properties. Also, it supports the immune system by reducing inflammation and increasing mast cell production. Tulasi has been used for centuries to treat a variety of disorders stemming from inflammation. Other health benefits include antipyretic (fever reducing), analgesic (pain reducing), and antioxidant properties.

Haridra (Curcuma longa): Haridra, also commonly known as turmeric, has been used for centuries in Asia to treat inflammatory diseases. Studies increasingly support the use of Haridra as a powerful anti-inflammatory. It may help fight infections and some cancers since it is also a powerful antioxidant that scavenges the body, eradicating free radicals that are known to cause damage to the cell membrane. As a result, Haridra may have beneficial therapeutic effects for BPH by reducing inflammation of the prostate gland. It may also reducde the risk of prostate cancer through its antioxidant activity.

Amalaki (Phyllanthus emblica): Amalaki is a tree indigenous to tropical regions of Southeast Asia. It produces gooseberries, which have been used traditionally to strengthen the immune system. They have also been shown to have potent tumor-inhibiting properties against a variety of cancers.

Ashwagandha (Withania somnifera): Ashwagandha is a potent adaptogenic herb that provides stress relieving properties. It has been particularly successful at improving infertility in men whose infertility is related to stress. As an adaptogen that supports the body's functions as a whole, Ashwagandha also supports prostate health by balancing sex hormones.

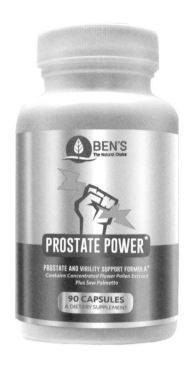

SUPPLEMENT FACTS
Serving Size: 1 Capsule
Serving Per Container: 90 Capsules

Ingredients	Amount Per Serving
Rye (Flower Pollen) Extract (Secale Cereale =L.) (Standardized Saw Palmetto Extract 45% PE)	213mg
Saw Palmetto (fruit) (Serenoa Repens L.) (Standardized Saw Palmetto Extract 45% PE)	213mg
Boron Glycine Complex 10% (Albion)	10mg

Daily Value (DV) of core ingredients not established.
Other Ingredients: Maltodextrin, Microcrystalline, Cellulose, Silicon Dioxide, Calcium Stearate, Monocalcium Phosphate, Gum Arabic, Rice Flour, Gelatin, Purified Water.

SUMMARY:

Ben's Prostate Power is a clinically formulated complex of nutrients that combines a pure rye flower pollen extract with 45% saw palmetto berry extract plus a boron chelate. It was formulated to reduce the urinary symptoms from BPH and prostatitis by reducing inflammation and shrinking the prostate gland. In our own patient reports, we have discovered this combination to add a powerful symptom alleviator when combined with Ben's Total Health for the Prostate and Ben's Prostate Healer Tincture.

A 2003 study conducted at the National Center for Natural Products Research, Research Institute of Pharmaceutical Sciences, University of Mississippi reviewed the existing literature on the use of flower pollen extract, as well as 45% saw palmetto berry. The researchers were interested in whether flower pollen extract provides symptomatic relief from lower urinary tract symptoms (LUTS). They concluded that rye pollen extract is a safe, effective, natural supplement for the relief of LUTS and improves quality-of-life for men with BPH and prostatitis. These effects are particularly so when the extract is used in combination with other dietary supplements, such as saw palmetto berry, or for men who prefer to go the pharmaceutical route, in combination with medications. The researchers admit uncertainty about how rye flower pollen extract works to reduce symptoms but suggest that it may be the result of an anti-inflammatory effect.

Numerous studies have arrived at similar conclusions about flower pollen extract and saw palmetto berry: significant reduction in symptoms and improvement in being able to empty the bladder completely. In some of the studies I have reviewed, men also reported an increase in semen production over the longer term, which persisted as long as they continued to take this combination.

ACTIVE INGREDIENTS:

Rye Flower Pollen Extract: Soothes and tones smooth muscles of bladder and urethra to reduce LUTS, strong anti-inflammatory, and also antiproliferative effects, meaning inhibits cellular proliferation of the prostate that contributes to BPH.

Saw Palmetto Berry: Contains Beta-Sitosterol, which inhibits the conversion of testosterone to DHT by inhibiting 5 alpha-reductase, the enzyme that would cause the conversion. As a result, it inhibits growth of the prostate and perhaps shrinks it, while also improving urinary symptoms.

Boron Glycine Complex: An important trace mineral, boron improves the body's use of estrogen, testosterone, and vitamin D, and thereby, importantly restoring male to female hormone balance. It also reduces inflammation, supports the immune system, boosts absorption of magnesium, and may have anti-carcinogenic properties.

ADDITIONAL NOTES:

The three active ingredients in Ben's Prostate Power are formulated to work synergistically to not only improve the symptoms of BPH and prostatitis, but also to address the causes of these symptoms: inflammation and prostate cell proliferation.

PROSTATE SUPPLEMENTS

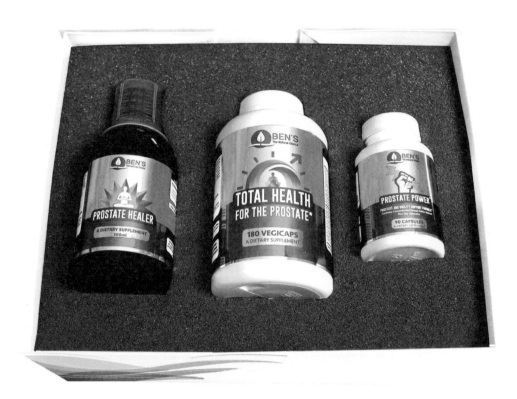

SUMMARY:

Ben's Prostate Health Program is a combination of three of the most effective supplements for prostate health: Ben's Total Health for the Prostate, Ben's Prostate Healer, and Ben's Prostate Power to provide comprehensive symptom reduction that fights diseases of the prostate, including BPH and prostatitis at the root causes. This complete program is not just a collection of beneficial ingredients. It is a clinically formulated bio-optimized complex of nutrients that work synergistically to combat symptoms and the disease process together. All the active ingredients listed above for each of these products are included in Ben's Prostate Health Program at the same potent doses, using the same quality ingredients and preparation methods.

PROSTATE SUPPLEMENTS

A combination of 3 of the most effective supplements for prostate health in the world. Exactly what you need to restore your prostate health, delivered straight to your door, every month. Each one is designed to work synergistically together while addressing different elements of prostate disease.

Together they help restore and maintain optimal prostate health, shrink the prostate gland, alleviate symptoms, lower PSA scores and clear out urinary, bladder and prostate infections.

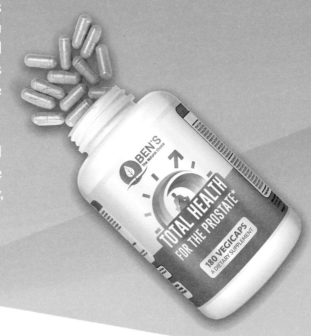

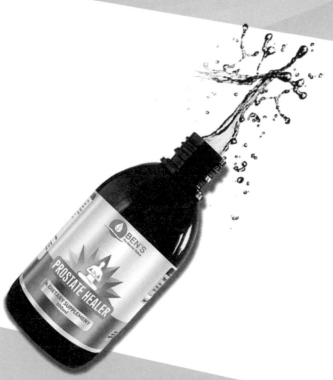

MORE POWERFUL & MORE EFFECTIVE

Different nutrients, compounds and ingredients need to be prepared in different ways to ensure maximum bioavailability and efficacy. All herbs are cold pressed and preserved in alcohol. Minerals are chelated with amino acids. Vitamins are natural, not synthetic. By creating a program of 3 supplements, you can have different preparations and different approaches, allowing you to maximize the potency and efficacy of each individual supplement.

BENEFITS & BONUSES

Being on the Prostate Health program has advantages over simply buying all 3 products individually, not least of all is a better price. But you also receive additional free seasonal supplements every few months that help you maintain general, mental and sexual health. You also get free upgraded shipping on each months shipment, and free access to the VIP content library that contains special reports, videos and exclusive content that is only for program members.

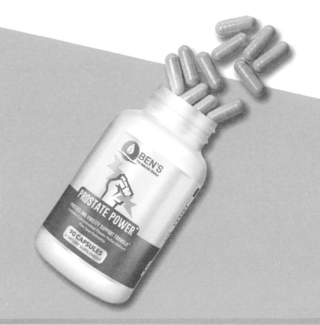

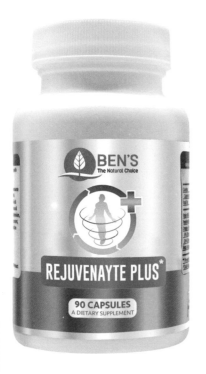

SUPPLEMENT FACTS

Serving Size: 3 Capsules
Serving Per Container: 30 Capsules

Ingredients	% Daily Value	Amount Per Serving
Green Tea (Leaf)	N/A	500mg
Cloves 4:1	N/A	400mg
Pomegranate Extract 4:1	N/A	200mg
Japanese Sophora (Quercitin)	N/A	200mg
Tumeric Curcumin	N/A	200mg
DHEA	N/A	50mg
Black Pepper (Peppercorns)	N/A	10mg

** = Daily Value (DV) has not been established.

SUMMARY:

Rejuvenayte Plus is a unique anti-prostate-cancer and quality-of-life enhancing supplement. It has the added benefits of supporting cognitive functioning and preventing age-related cognitive decline.

ACTIVE INGREDIENTS:

Green Tea Leaf (98% Polyphenols, 50% EGCG [epigallocatechin gallate]): Powerful antioxidant that prevents free radical damage and protects against cancer by promoting cancer cell death and inhibiting cancer cell proliferation. Also protects DNA, which protects against cancer. Boosts immune system and reduces inflammation. Green Tea Leaf polyphenols are potent support for prostate cancer health.

Clove: The 5th most powerful antioxidant in nature, preventing free radical damage and protecting against cancer by promoting cancer cell death and inhibiting cancer cell proliferation. Strong support for the immune system and anti-inflammatory.

Pomegranate (Ellagic Acid): A strong antioxidant and anti-cancer nutrient.

Japanese Sophora Flower Buds (Quercetin): A natural antioxidant that has been shown to relieve symptoms of prostatitis and BPH while also promoting cellular health in general.

Turmeric (Curcuma longa): Used for centuries in Asia to treat inflammation. Studies increasingly support the use of Turmeric as a powerful anti-inflammatory. It may help fight infections and some cancers since it is also a powerful antioxidant that scavenges the body, eradicating free radicals that are known to cause damage to cell membranes. As a result, Turmeric may have beneficial therapeutic effects for BPH by not only reducing inflammation of the prostate gland but also reducing the risk of prostate cancer through its antioxidant activity.

DHEA: With aging, levels of dehydroepiandrosterone (DHEA) decrease, which may be linked to the development of ED. Supplementing with DHEA may reverse this process. Also helps numerous functions across the body to maintain optimal physical health.

Black Pepper (Peppercorns, organic): Enhances the bioavailability and potency of several of the herbs in this Rejuvenayte Plus formulation, particularly Turmeric.

ADDITIONAL BENEFITS

Cloves have strong anti-microbial properties. Japanese Sophora Flower Buds have been shown to increase stamina and improve cardiovascular health.

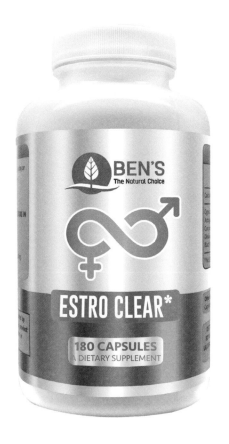

SUPPLEMENT FACTS
Serving Size: 6 Capsules
Serving Per Container: 30 Capsules

Ingredients	% Daily Value	Amount Per Serving
Calcium D Glucarate	99%	985mg
Cyperus Extract 10:1	N/A	1000mg
Astragalus 50% Polysaccharides	N/A	500mg
Curcuma Zedoaria Extract 10:1	N/A	500mg
Diindolylmethane (DIM) 98%	N/A	200mg
Organic Black Peppercorn	N/A	10mg

** = Daily Value (DV) has not been established.

SUMMARY:

Ben's Estro-Clear is formulated to flush excess estrogen and therefore restore the normal hormone balance. Many men in the US and UK now suffer from what is referred to as estrogen dominance, which can cause female pattern fat distribution, including breast tissue. Estrogen dominant men may lose their sense of physical stamina and strength. To add insult to injury, fat cells actually produce estrogen, creating a vicious cycle. Estrogen dominance also causes an increase in thyroid-binding globulin, which can result in hypothyroidism, which again, may cause weight gain and the worsening cycle of estrogen dominance. In recent years, this pattern has become defined as the male version of menopause and has been referred to as "andropause."

Conventional medicine has long paid little attention to andropause and estrogen dominance in men. They neither understood the mechanisms and consequences, nor did they have any particular concern to treat them—the old refrain: "just a product of aging." At best, men might get a new drug prescription that might alleviate some of the urinary symptoms from BPH, but with the corresponding side effects that these drugs cause.

Not surprisingly, men who were affected by andropause fell in line with their doctors in thinking these symptoms were an inevitable part of aging. As with prostate disease, estrogen dominance and andropause are not inevitable. Along with the diet and lifestyle changes that are crucial for changing this pattern, Ben's Estro Clear will supplement these positive changes, clearing out excess estrogen and restoring your normal male hormone balance, which means regaining your healthy masculine traits (burning excess fat around the chest and middle, and strengthening muscle tone).

ACTIVE INGREDIENTS:

Calcium Carbonate Glucarate: Aids in the body's excretion of used hormones before they can be reabsorbed. You might think of it as a scavenger for excess hormones and toxins. Flushing excess estrogen is key for prostate health. While not considered to be an essential recommended daily nutrient, perhaps because the body makes small amounts of Calcium Carbonate Glucarate, low levels of this compound have been correlated with higher levels of Beta-glucuronidase. Elevated Beta-glucuronidase levels have been shown to be a risk factor for cancer, especially hormone-related cancers like prostate and breast cancers.

The daily dosage of Calcium Carbonate Glucarate in Ben's Estro Clear is equivalent to the phytonutrient activity found in 160 pounds of fresh fruits and vegetables.
New research has shown that Calcium Carbonate Glucarate is just as effective as Tamoxifen in treating estrogen dominance and could be just as effective in preventing cancer as Tamoxifen, but with none of the side-effects.

Cyperus: Natural aromatase reducers that can reduce estradiol level. Aromatase inhibitors prevent the male body from converting testosterone into estrogen.

Astragalus: A perennial flowering plant prevalent in northern China, Mongolia, and Korea with long history of medicinal use to increase boost the immune system, metabolism, stamina, strength, and vitality. Astragalus continues to be widely used in Traditional Chinese Medicine, often combined with other herbs. Astragalus works by improving communication between the hormones and hormone-regulating chemicals, thereby supporting a normal balance.

Curcuma zedoaria: A member of the Curcuma family, and turmeric, this rhizome has strong anti-inflammatory properties.

Diindoylymethane (DIM): A component of Indole-3-carbinol (I3C) found in members of the Brassica family, most notably broccoli, kale, and cauliflower. It has potent effects on estrogen metabolism and is able to keep the body relatively balanced (by preventing either drastic increases or decreases in estrogen). In small amounts, it can inhibit the aromatase enzyme (and prevent conversion of testosterone into estrogen), and it can act on more potent forms of estrogen and convert them into less potent forms. This conversion reduces the overall effects of estrogen in the body. DIM also exerts numerous anti-carcinogenic (anti-cancer) effects in the body and is one of the reasons this vegetable family is considered to be so healthy.

Black Pepper (Peppercorn, organic): Enhances the bioavailability and potency of several of the herbs in this Estro Clear formulation, particularly Curcuma zedoaria.

ADDITIONAL BENEFITS:

Calcium Carbonate Glucarate has also been shown to be beneficial in detoxifying or ridding carcinogens from the body, making it a beneficial nutrient to potentially reduce the risk of prostate cancer. As toxin exposure continues to increase in the world we live in today, excreting toxins becomes increasing important.

In Asia, Cyperus has been known for centuries to balance Chi (the human energy force). Additional benefits of Astragulus include protective properties for the liver, kidneys and urinary system, as well as being rich in antioxidants, and having anti-inflammatory properties. It also may have energy-boosting qualities.

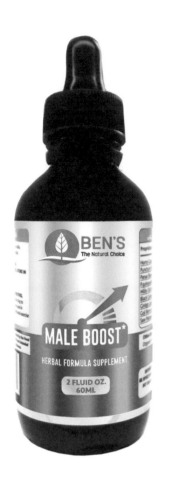

SUPPLEMENT FACTS
Serving Size: 1/2 Teaspoon
Serving Per Container: 90

Ingredients (Proprietary Blend)

Flowering Barrenwort (Epimedium Brevicorum)

Puncture Vine Seed (Trinbulus Terristris)

Panax Blend (mixture of P. Gineseng, P. Notoginseng & P. Quinquefolius)

Milky Oat Seed (Avena Sativa)

Black Cohosh Root (Actea/Cimicifuga Racemosa)

Ginkgo Leaf (Ginkgo Biloba)

Goji Berry (Lycium Chinesis)

Saw Palmetto Berry (Serenoa Serrulata)

SUMMARY:

Ben's Male Boost Tincture is formulated to naturally boost your sexual energy and stamina, increase libido, and reverse ED. As a tincture, Male Boost is a proprietary blend of 10 concentrated phytonutrients that have multiple actions on the sexual and immune systems, as well as toning and calming effects on the nervous system, helping to provide an overall sense of well-being. The herbs in Ben's Male Boost Tincture have been shown to increase testosterone and nitric oxide levels, leading to stronger erections. It also may help your body to produce more semen.

PROSTATE SUPPLEMENTS

ACTIVE INGREDIENTS:

Puncture Vine Weed (Tribulus terristris): With aging, levels of dehydroepiandrosterone (DHEA) decrease, which may be linked to the development of ED. Puncture vine weed has been shown to increase DHEA, thereby enhancing erection. Other studies suggest that puncture vine weed may also increase nitric oxide (NO), which is critical for a strong erection.

Flowering Barrenwort (Epimedium brevicorum): Has been used for centuries in Traditional Chinese Medicine to treat ED for the active phytonutrient Icarin. Lab studies show that horny goat weed has an "erectogenic" effect, perhaps from an increase in NO production.

Panax Ginseng Root (Chinese ginseng) & Panax Quinquefolius Root (American ginseng): Another herb that has a rich history in Traditional Chinese Medicine, ginseng is a strong adaptogenic herb that has been used for several thousand years to tone and restore all systems of the body and thereby promote health and well-being. These adaptogenic properties are also thought to enhance physical performance, including sexual stamina. Lab studies have shown that it may improve production of NO, thereby strengthening erections.

Milky Oat Seed (Aveena sativa): Thought to improve sexual function and premature ejaculation by its "nervine" or calming effects.

Black Cohosh Root (Actea/Cimicifuga racemosa): Anti-depressant, immune strengthening, and anti-inflammatory properties to shrink prostate with its negative effect on erectile function.

Ginkgo Leaf (Ginkgo biloba): Powerful antioxidant that naturally supports the free radical fighting abilities of the body to fight against oxidative stress and prevent cell damage.

Goji Berry (Lycium chinesis): Strong anti-oxidant and mood enhancer that promotes serenity and sleep quality. Also enhances physical performance.

Saw Palmetto Berry: Contains Beta-Sitosterol. As a result, it inhibits growth of the prostate and perhaps shrinks it, while also improving LUTS and ED.

ADDITIONAL NOTES:

Please note that Ben's Male Boost Tincture is NOT suitable if:

- You are advised not to engage sexual activity, such as with severe heart failure or unstable angina.
- You take medication specifically for disorders of libido.
- You take nitroglycerin, such as Nitro Advance®, among others.
- You take prescribed medicines for high or low blood pressure.
- You take anti-inflammatory drugs (NSAIDS), such as ibuprofen or Naproxen®, among others.
- You take ACE inhibitors or potassium-sparing diuretics.
- You experience dizziness especially when getting up and if you have low blood pressure.
- You have a genital herpes infection.
- You are under 18 years old.
- You exhibit sensitivity to one or more ingredients in Male Boost.

You will note that lycopene, nettles, star grass, and a whole host of other herbs are often touted as miracle cures for prostate disease, are not on my list of recommended nutrients. I have chosen to omit these ingredients because, while they may have some nutritional value in general, which I won't dispute, the effects of these nutrients on the prostate is either overhyped or not supported by solid scientific research.

LYCOPENE

There has been a very misleading but successful promotion regarding the benefits of lycopene, which is a by-product of cooking tomatoes. Some studies claim that by eating cooked tomatoes, you can improve prostate health, so much so that one study claimed the more pizza men ate, the more prostate health they achieved! This kind of pseudoscience is asinine. Many other dietary studies contradict this conclusion. Actual blood serum level studies of lycopene prove there is no correlation between lycopene levels and prostate health. Plus, no matter how how much tomato juice you drink or cooked tomatoes you eat, you won't raise lycopene levels. The tomatoes must be cooked in oil for lycopene to be absorbable.

NETTLE LEAF EXTRACT

Nettle leaf is another nutrient that is often promoted or sold as good for prostate health. The leaf is approximately 1% Beta-Sitosterol. The root has slightly more but not significantly so. This low percentage of Beta-Sitosterols means that it will never have a significant effect on your prostate health.

That said, nettle leaf is actually a secret super food. The dried leaf of nettle is 40% protein and is rich in a whole suite of vitamins including A, C, D, E, F, K, P. Furthermore, nettle leaf is rich in antioxidants as well as B vitamins, such as thiamine, riboflavin, niacin, and folate. Nettle also contains a high content of the trace minerals, including selenium, zinc, iron, and magnesium, not to mention boron, sodium, iodine, chromium, copper, and sulphur. Supplements don't provide all these nutrients, however. For these overall health benefits, it is best to eat nettles, such as soups or to drink nettle tea.

PROSTATE SUPPLEMENTS

PUMPKIN SEED OIL

Pumpkin seeds and pumpkin seed oil are a new trendy health food that while nutritious when you eat them, provide negligible benefits when included in a supplement. Pumpkin seeds contain a variety of trace minerals, two of which are especially healthy for the prostate: selenium and zinc. They also are rich in vitamin E. But when the oil of pumpkin seeds is extracted into supplement form, the quantity of these active ingredients is too little to be beneficial. You would have to eat one and a half pounds of pumpkin seeds to get a clinically significant dose of selenium, for instance. If you look at a bottle of pumpkin seed extract in supplement form, you will find that the daily dose is about 1000 mg, which is clinically insignificant. Also, when you consider that the weight of a single pumpkin seed is about 750 mg, then with a 1000 mg supplement dose, all you are consuming is the equivalent of just over 1 seed a day. If you want the health benefits of pumpkin seeds, my advice is to eat them raw in salads.

HOW MANY SUPPLEMENTS IS ENOUGH

As I mentioned at the beginning of this section on supplements, many people are used to thinking that pills and capsules are pharmaceuticals or work like them, so some real hesitation arises when people start thinking about taking them. The first thought is often: what side effects am I going to have to deal with? The second thought is often along the lines of: how many do I have to take?

Most people are well aware that drugs have side effects and so often, the more you take, the more the side effects and the more dangerous those interactions become. The understandable knee jerk reaction is I don't want to take too many pills. It is important to understand, however, that dietary supplements and pharmaceutical medications are not the same.

I am repeating here something I said at the introduction to this section because it cannot be emphasized enough: dietary supplements are not magic pills that miraculously undo disease while you go on living a life that contributes to it. Dietary supplements work synergistically with a healthy lifestyle, including proper diet, exercise, as well as stress and overload management. Their "mechanisms of action" are also not singularly targeted, like drugs are, so when adding dietary supplements to our lives, we need to first change our mindset from the one that we have about pharmaceuticals.

Secondly, dietary supplements rarely have side effects and then typically only if you happen to be allergic to one of the ingredients. It is a good idea to read the labels to make sure that any supplement you are about to purchase does not contain ingredients you are allergic to. Even on the rare occasion that a person experiences a side effect to a dietary supplement, it is usually fairly innocuous, like a skin rash or an upset stomach. But these symptoms should be paid attention to and typically go away as soon as you stop taking the supplements. It is important to remember that dietary supplements are concentrated forms of foods or plants that we in the modern world no longer consider to be a regular part of our diet, but which are food nonetheless.

The objective of taking dietary supplements is to boost the variety and amount of your daily nutrient intake, and by this I am clearly not referring to carbs, proteins, and fats, though there are some dietary supplements that balance out healthy fats for our typically unhealthy fatty acid balance. But I won't go into the details of all that here. The point I want to emphasize is that dietary supplements should be taken with an appreciation for the nutrient value they are adding. So, taking this supplement and that supplement is not the same as taking this drug and that drug. You might think of it simply as eating a greater variety of highly nutritious food—provided you are taking good quality nutrients, which I discussed earlier in this chapter.

Then there is the dread of taking all those pills and capsules. Tinctures make this dread about taking a handful of pills a little more varied. And, if you get into the habit of adding supplements to your daily regimen, very soon it becomes an old habit—a healthy one. Some people begin, for instance, by taking only the Ben's Prostate Health Program. It's a good start and a comprehensive set of 3 supplements that work together. Then add other supplements a step at a time. Doing this stepping up method allows you to see how each supplement is working for you.

So, to the first question: how many capsules should you take? Well, the answer to this question is up to you, of course. Because dietary supplements are food, the more variety you take, the more nourishment you are giving your body, boosting your health along the way. You might turn this question to a plate of food by asking, if I eat spinach do I also need carrots? The answer is the more variety you have, the better it is for your health. The real limitations are about getting into this adding nutrient value mindset, habit, and considering what you can afford.

On affordability, if I have heard it once I have heard it more times than I can count that people think skimping on price will save them money. Well, perhaps, in that one short moment. But across the board, when it comes to food and supplements, dollars spent now are healthcare dollars saved later. Spending that extra percentage at the grocery counter for organic produce and on supplements that don't skimp on quality may save you thousands of dollars down the road on medical bills.

If cost is an issue, and it is for many people, look for supplements that are of the highest quality but that also contain a number of nutrients in one formulation. That way you are not spending as many dollars on bottle after bottle of supplement. This also means fewer pills or capsules to pop into your mouth each day—if you are not a pill person. The other thing is to ask for reliable advice on what supplements you can reasonably leave out. If you ever have questions about Ben's supplements, which ones, how many, which to prioritize and which ones to wait on, email us. Again, make sure to provide as much information as possible so that we can steer you in the right direction. We are glad to help.

Hardly a day passes that I do not receive at least one unsolicited comment from a customer. Every man is individual and reacts differently. I am not suggesting that every man who reads this guide will feel the same in a year. Nor am I saying that any man who takes my supplements will necessarily have the same experience. Every person's set of circumstances, issues, and needs are different, as well as responses to the program I recommend in this guide. What I can tell you is that there is no better way to improve the health of your prostate naturally, and your overall health.

SUPPLEMENTS FOR OTHER CONDITIONS

Since this guide is about prostate disease, I do not go into detail discussing supplements for other chronic conditions. That said, many men with prostate disease also suffer from other chronic conditions as well. Ben's Natural Health addresses a variety of other conditions, especially insulin resistance, metabolic syndrome, prediabetes, and diabetes. If you have other medical problems, please contact us and we will be happy to help. I can be reached at: support@bensnaturalhealth.com

EXCEPTIONAL PRODUCTS WITH THE FINEST QUALITY CONTROL

While it is possible to get many of supplements that I recommend from other manufacturers in different formulations, and, as I have indicated, it is important for you to experience for yourself whether our formulations are right for you, I want you to know before purchasing even one of Ben's supplements the strict guidelines that we follow to ensure finest quality control. You should know about the manufacturing practices of any dietary supplement producer. And, you should expect nothing less than exceptional bio-optimized products for your health.

Ben's Natural Health operates stringent quality control, even greater than required by the FDA (Food and Drug Administration). Our factory is a CGMP (current good manufacturing practice regulations) manufacturing facility, which is certified under 21 CRF Part III (a code of regulations for food and drug manufacturers). We are a registered facility with the FDA.

All our processing and manufacturing is done in isolated production rooms (clean rooms) to prevent any cross contamination of ingredients and products. Our comprehensive, exacting standard operating procedures determine every facet of the process.

Ben's Natural Health testing protocols are established utilizing an NSF (National Science Foundation) designed hazard analysis program. Even where the risk is very low, every raw material is tested using USP (United States Pharmacopeia) and/or AHPA (American Herbal Products Association) recommended standards. USP standards are used to demonstrate identity, strength, purity, and quality for medicines, dietary supplements, and food ingredients. As a result, we guarantee that all our botanicals are radiation free. Our monitoring program ensures that no radiation has been used in the sterilization of our botanicals. When sterilization is needed, we use a dry steam technology or other non-destructive technologies.

In accordance with the most stringent of FDA protocols, we conduct, in-house, 100% testing using USP method 1119 Near-Infrared spectroscopy, a scientific process that uses chemometric models to identify all raw materials. Our reference standards are third-party laboratory-verified, certifying their validity. This hand selected, third-party laboratory holds the international ISO 17025 certificate, which certifies the competence of lab testing.

We conduct regular audits of our outside laboratory partners. Environmental testing for microbiological bio-burden hazards is an integral part of Ben's testing program. Introduction of microbial adulterants during holding or processing is monitored utilizing USP Method 1116 (the most recommended method to test for contaminants) for continued evaluation of microbial limits in controlled areas. This method was adopted by Ben's voluntarily from the pharmaceutical codes. Dietary supplement regulations do not require this, but we believe it is imperative for quality.

Ben's Natural Health has also developed a program utilizing spectroscopy USP method 1119 to establish chemometric models of finished products. These testing models are then used to assure that each product meets all intended identity, strength, and composition specifications unique to the finished product batch. Finally, every finished batch is tested again for microbial adulteration, thus assuring that every batch meets our purity standards.

Ben's Natural Health maintains a robust hazard analysis program that reviews the potential for risks associated with each of our manufacturers of ingredients following NSF guidelines. Mitigations describe how a risk level is reduced by the design of our quality systems. Immediate precautions are designed to block hazards in normal conditions. Also included in these mitigations are at least one upstream and one downstream protection to block the potential hazard from entering the processing chain. These mitigations are ingredient-specific and are added to each ingredient specification sheet, assuring that each time that ingredient is received it is reviewed and tested for its unique hazard(s).

All ingredients have risks and require systems to block sources of contaminants. We do not rely on our nutrient supplier for your safety. Risks, such as radiation contamination, heavy metals, E. coli, salmonella, staph, dangerous spores, and economic adulteration, are monitored by our rigorous testing methodology. By identifying such risks ahead of time, the mitigation process enables us to block these hazards.

The Ben's Natural Health procurement team is continually seeking the purest ingredients from the finest suppliers around the globe, so that we can provide all our customers quality and assurance for making the right changes to a better life.

We promise you only the very best for your health!

PART 4:

Ben's Last Words
Of Wisdom

WHAT TO DO WHEN YOU DON'T SEEM TO BE IMPROVING

The program that I have outlined for you requires substantial changes: by improving diet and adding exercise, managing stress, reducing toxin exposure, and supplementing with dietary supplements. Very often, when men report that they are not improving, it is because they have not made the sufficient changes in all these areas. But it is also true that some men who follow these recommendations religiously and take the supplements I recommend here, continue to experience symptoms, and their PSA levels continue to increase over an extended period.

If you find yourself in this situation, then it may be that you do, in fact, have prostate cancer. Remember please that having a prostate cancer diagnosis is not a death sentence. Most prostate cancers are contained to the prostate and very slow growing, and many men live with this diagnosis for years without any problem. What these men die of is not prostate cancer.

The question is what do you do if your disease worsens and you develop prostate cancer? If you wish to avoid biopsy and subsequent invasive treatments, there is certainly a strong argument for taking a more rigorous approach to diet and lifestyle and also taking additional supplements. If you do have prostate cancer, then it is important to know if it is localized or aggressive and potentially life-threatening. Following these diet and lifestyle changes will not hurt you, even if you have an aggressive form of prostate cancer and choose conventional medical intervention. These changes can only boost your body's capacity to heal.

The question to consider always when confronted with invasive treatments for BPH and localized prostate cancer is the quality of your life as a result of the treatment(s). Incontinence and impotence are not fun. Studies over the last 20 years consistently show that your life expectancy is not improved by any one or more invasive treatments for these conditions.

One very viable consideration, though it is quite expensive and not covered by insurance is an APCRA screening, which I discussed in Part 1. A naturopathic physician who is also a professor of urology performs APCRA screenings on our patients in my Arizona clinic. Generally, an APCRA screening will reveal not only whether you have prostate cancer, but it will also indicate what kind of prostate cancer it is, how aggressive, and if it is likely to become life threatening.

If your PSA continues to rise and cancer is in question, and if you can afford my APCRA screening, I strongly recommend it. It will provide the most comprehensive information about the cancer and address the stress you may have about what is going on inside your prostate—all without adding the risk of having a biopsy. If this is something that you would like to know more about, please feel free to email us at support@bensnaturalhealth.com or give us a phone call on 1-888-868-3554.

SITTING ON THE FENCE

It is not surprising that many men are uncertain about whether to trust mainstream medicine or a more natural approach such as the one I have outlined in this guide. As a result of this ambivalence, many opt to sit on the fence and go both ways—conventional and natural. Other men take go the natural route, all the while keeping one eye on the possibility of drugs, surgery, radiation, and so on, just in case this path does not work for them. There is nothing wrong with this "sitting on the fence" approach, especially since prostate disease tends to move at a glacial pace. Usually, there is plenty of time to determine whether you can avoid the harsher mainstream treatments. But there are several dangers to sitting on the fence that are good to bear in mind.

The first has to do with level of commitment. If at the back of his mind, a man thinks, Well, if supplements don't work, I still have the medical options, he is likely to be far less committed to the natural route. This stance is understandable. After all, making such radical lifestyle changes can be one hell of an effort for many people.

If, on the other hand, a man is fully committed to the natural route, he will go the extra mile to make every possible change to maximize his chance of improving the health of his prostate. My concern for men who may be inclined to sit on the fence is that doing so can limit commitment to the work of making the necessary diet and lifestyle changes. There is always the possibility of one foot out the door of these changes when the work of it gets to be too demanding. To go the natural route, you must be "all in" or it won't work.

The second danger is a little subtler and has to do with taking both routes simultaneously. Drugs reduce symptoms and can mask a worsening condition. That means you may not get signals from your body about whether your diet and lifestyle efforts are working. You become instead more dependent on bio-chemical measurements that the doctor is likewise relying on. This is not to say that these "biomarkers" are not helpful. Some of them give us an additional bit of information about how the prostate is functioning, and we also need to give a good deal of attention to how we are feeling: symptoms, energy, sexual drive and function, and so on.

Third, there are the problems associated with the negative impact that some conventional medical treatments have on your immune system. In fact, strengthening your immune system to improve your health and that of your prostate is a major whole objective of improving nutrition and lifestyle. The natural approach boosts the body's own functions at fighting disease. As a result, in sitting on the fence, you could be pulling in two opposing directions.

Finally, and not least, some of the damage that can occur with conventional medical treatment is irreparable. I receive e-mails from unhappy men every day who complain about the consequences of one or other treatment, asking if there is a way to reverse it. It pains me when I have to say to them, "Sorry, that damage is irreversible." Most of those cries for help seem to come from men who have lost the ability to have sex or who have become incontinent.

Sitting on the fence is an understandable approach to increase my odds. In fact, it does little to help your odds. The only way to take on this natural approach is to do so with 100% commitment. Sure, you may have to go at it one step at a time, but without 100% commitment, your odds for improving the health of your prostate are dramatically reduced.

WHY PROSTATE CANCER REOCCURS AFTER MAINSTREAM TREATMENT

One of the most common problems for patients who undergo conventional medical treatment for prostate cancer is recurrence. Many men are given to think they have beaten their cancer through a combination of hormone treatments, radiation, and surgery, only to find a few years later that tumors have spread into nearby organs. Though research is starting to point to markers of inflammation and hormone imbalances as I have discussed in this guide, modern medicine, by and large, continues to treat the symptoms and not the cause. And, as I've emphasized, even when research clearly points to hormone imbalances and not excess testosterone, clinical physicians keep trying to lower testosterone!

For someone who sees disease through a holistic lens, cancer is a symptom of an underlying problem within the body's ecosystem. Disease occurs because the balance that keeps the body healthy is out of whack. The system is stressed, and normal functions begin to break down. Without a solid understanding of the body as a balance of interactions and functions, and without therefore treating underlying imbalances, modern medicine will never eliminate the underlying cause of cancer. What that means for you and me as potential patients of this medical approach is that, in the case of prostate cancer, even after becoming "cancer-free" through conventional therapies, you are still at risk of developing prostate cancer again—because those treatments don't get at the cause!

You might think of it like this: suppose there is a dam holding back a large body of water. From the outside, all seems to be going well. The water is behind the dam wall. One day, water starts leaking through. In the world of conventional medicine, the approach would be to go to the leak and put a patch over it to eliminate the water from flooding the valley below.

But the problem isn't the water leaking through the dam; the problem is the structural integrity of the dam combined with the volume of water behind the dam. Once erected, someone needed to be there to watch what the dam could handle given the water levels. This is a situation akin to the "too much" scenario that our bodies face within our modern lives—bad food, toxins, stress, and so on, coupled the "not enough" scenario—nutrients, exercise, restoration. Too much water behind the dam now stresses the strength of the dam. Leaks in the dam are a sign that it is reaching capacity. Patching the leak will only lead to more leaks later because the source of the problem hasn't been addressed.

The same is true with prostate cancer. The cause of the cancer needs to be addressed and rectified. The best way to do that is via changes in diet and lifestyle with the addition of supplements to turbo-charge the body's own functions. Unless you boost the body's health-generating and immune system functions, then you're just chasing symptoms—skipping from one dam leak to another.

The cancer is the symptom, not the cause. I know it can be hard to wrap our minds around this perspective, but we need to rewire how we think of disease. Disease is a symptom of systems breakdown.

Also, here is an equally difficult piece of information to wrap our minds around: just because you remove the prostate for prostate cancer does not mean you will not have prostate cancer again. Sure, the prostate has been removed, but the problem of the cancer is still at work in the body. It's kind of like fire. Once the flame is going, there is fire as long as the conditions are right to support it. You can take the majority of the logs out of the fire place and still have fire burning in there. If you have aggressive prostate cancer and choose to have the prostate removed, the only hope for not having recurrence is to make drastic changes to diet and lifestyle so as not to feed the cancer fire, and to boost your body's functions with nutrient-packed dietary supplements.

As to the question of how one attempts to eliminate the cause in the first place? I hope I have shown you plenty of evidence in this guide. Work to improve your diet, reduce stress and toxin overload, and add exercise and dietary supplements. This lifestyle regimen is a comprehensive way to support the body in being healthy and preventing disease, and in healing itself if or when disease comes knocking, particularly as we age.

AN AFTERWORD: YOU DON'T HAVE TO DO THIS ON YOUR OWN

First of all, congratulations on reading this guide from start to finish! The information in this book on diseases of the prostate is second to none. I don't know of a more comprehensive guide out there, informed by years of research translated to make it accessible and informative for men trying to prevent or reverse prostate disease. Reading this guide is just the beginning of your journey to better prostate health.

I won't lie to you: getting healthy can be HARD WORK, but it is worth it. A longer, richer, more enjoyable life will be your reward. The important thing to know is that you are not alone. You are now part of a large community of informed men who are committed to overcoming prostate disease.

I invite you to reach out to me or any member of the community for support anytime you need. You can find us on YouTube, join the conversation on Facebook—where I post every day and you can message me—or email me. Our Facebook page is also a great place to find inspiration from men who have been exactly where you may be now and a great way to interact with the community. And there are tons of great personal stories, recipes, and tips and tricks that men post who are either fighting the same battles that you are or have already won their war on prostate disease! Speaking of recipes, check out the blogs I run that will inspire you with tasty recipes to stay on track with your new diet. And, the Prostate Health Association is available when you purchase Ben's Total Health for the Prostate. You can learn more about this on my website: www.bensnaturalhealth.com.

If you ever get stuck, lose motivation or need advice or support, or simply want some good ideas for a healthy recipe, then I personally want you to know that this community is here to help. The number and quality of resources available to you are staggering: daily and weekly email newsletters. I also print an in-depth, full-color, monthly magazine that has exclusive content and research breakdowns that I send for free to VIP subscribers. If you haven't yet signed up for emails, do so to automatically subscribe to the monthly journal. At Ben's Natural Health, our aim is always to support a growing community of people who want to take back control of their health.

For men and women who are struggling with other chronic diseases, we are putting together programs similar to this one on prostate health. For instance, just recently I also finished writing a guide on reversing diabetes, entitled, How to Reverse Diabetes in Fast. Many people think that diabetes is a lifelong condition that cannot be undone, reversed, halted, or even cured. This view is off the mark. As with prostate disease, I have dedicated extensive research efforts on diabetes, and I think I'm a decade ahead of the curve. And let me tell you, with the approach I offer in my new guide, diabetes is done for!

You will recall from what I shared earlier that at one time, as a result of eating what I thought at the time to be healthy, I developed diabetes. The high carb diet that was all the rage in the 80s and 90s became my demise. But, using the same approach I had to prostate disease, I was able to cure my own diabetes in less than ninety days! How to Reverse Diabetes in Fast is a step-by-step guide detailing exactly how I overcame diabetes and how you can too!

I point you in the direction of all these resources that are always growing because I want you to know that you are not alone in this fight, so much so that if you are really struggling and need my advice or support, write to me anytime, any day, and I will get back to you. That's right, my team personally respond to almost 200 questions a day from customers and men who are concerned about their health. Our email address is: support@bensnaturalhealth.com

If you are not a technical person, we've got you covered too. Request a call and one of my personally trained support consultants will telephone you at your convenience, and for free, to advise you on your health. There is a whole community just waiting here for you. All you have to do is reach out and become part of the Million-Man Prostate Health Revolution!

Finally, I want to thank you for reading this guide and joining the growing community of men taking the steps necessary to a fuller, healthier life!

Here's to your health!

Ben Ong

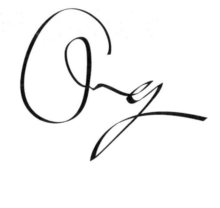

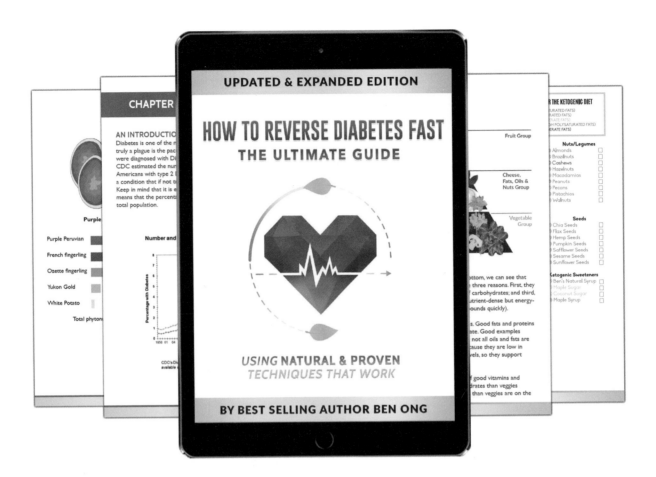

HOW TO REVERSE DIABETES FAST is a comprehensive, easy-to-follow ebook and guide on how you can lose weight, lower your blood sugar, and reverse type 2 diabetes using 100% natural methods.

Using the latest peer-reviewed, scientific research, this guide will look into what exactly causes diabetes; the personal and financial costs; why type 2 diabetes around the world is on the rise; why many drugs used to manage diabetes will do more harm for you than good; and how you can naturally reverse diabetes.

The guide lays out an evidence-based approach to reversing diabetes, backed by independent academic, medical and charitable organizations as well as a wealth of peer-reviewed research. This digital ebook lays out an easy, step-by-step plan that will help you reverse your type 2 diabetes in 90 days without drugs, surgery or side effects.

Note: "How To Reverse Diabetes" is only available as a digital ebook.

VISIT WWW.BENSDIABETES.COM FOR MORE INFORMATION

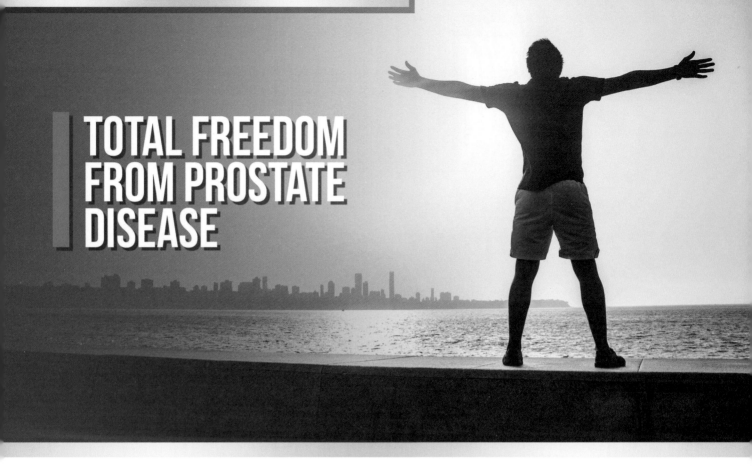
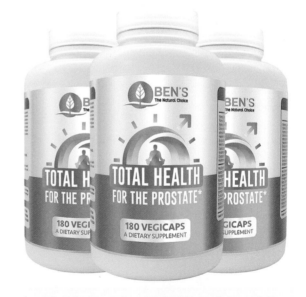
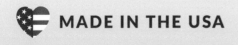
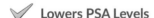

APPENDIX : RESEARCH ON TESTOSTERONE

This appendix is a summary of all of the research on the role of testosterone in prostate health, prostate enlargement, and prostate cancer. Over the course of many years, and many studies my clinical nutrition team and I have become convinced that high testosterone levels are not the cause of prostate disease, a fact that the medical establishment is only now catching up to. If you read through this appendix you will see that for decades the research has shown that low testosterone, not high testosterone, is a problem and that it is, in fact, dihydrotestosterone and estrogen that are responsible for many of your prostate problems.

There are four things to note about this appendix.

Firstly, this document stands separately from the book as a whole.

Secondly, this is a summary of many different studies and so for reasons one and two, the referencing system is slightly different from the rest of the book. For the rest of the book, all references can be found in the references section. For this section, end-notes link each summary and conclusion concerning a study to the specific study, so that if you wish to read the study in full you are able to.

Thirdly, some of the studies cited in this appendix are unavailable because they are either not available in English or too old and do not exist on the internet. These references will be marked as (NETA) No English Translation Available, or (NDA) Not Digitally Available.

Finally, while this Appendix contains a vast number of studies it is not exhaustive and is only up to date at the time of the publication of this edition of my book. More studies can be found on my website and are frequently explained and discussed alongside prostate health in my email newsletters.

If any of the information is news to you or contradicts what you have previously been told by doctors or specialists, I would suggest you ask them how much of the research they have read. Because the weight of evidence in defense of testosterone is overwhelming.

TESTOSTERONE RESEARCH

A study conducted at the University of Washington in 1999 examined if androgen supplementation should be considered as a treatment to reduce the growth of prostate cancer. Their research pointed out that declining testosterone levels contribute to the growth of cancer and that supplementing low levels to increase testosterone levels could reduce cancer rates. This study pointed also to earlier studies showing that low testosterone levels in prostate cancer patients indicated a much worse prognosis. [1]

At the University of Witwatersrand in South Africa in 1997, researchers produced a study demonstrating that out of 122 patients, those with the highest levels of testosterone had the least aggressive tumors. These patients also lived the longest. In contrast, the patients with the lowest testosterone levels had far more aggressive tumor growth and died much sooner. The researchers concluded, "Low testosterone seems to result in a more aggressive disease and a poorer prognosis in advanced prostate cancer". [2]

At the Hubei Medical University in China in 1998, researchers studied men with BPH and prostate cancer. Their research noted "that serum testosterone in patients with BPH and PCA [prostate cancer] was lower than that of the healthy control group," and further, "...the ratio of testosterone-to-estradiol is decreased with the rise of the age. The results suggested that the imbalance of serum sex hormones (i.e., falling testosterone and rising estrogen) was related to the pathogenesis of BPH and PCA". [3] This is the exact opposite of what was and to some degree still is the opinion of the medical establishment.

At the University of Vienna in 2000, five men with prostate cancer were compared to healthy controls. The men with cancer had decidedly lower testosterone levels than the healthy men. [4]

Another study conducted at the University of Vienna in 2001 showed that "patients with high Gleason score prostate cancer have lower testosterone levels." The men with the lowest Gleason scores and slowest growing malignancies had high testosterone levels averaging 4.1 ng/ml; the ones with the highest Gleason scores and fastest growing malignancies had low testosterone levels averaging only 2.8 ng/ml. The men with almost 50% higher testosterone levels fared much better. [5]

In a later study, the University of Vienna in 2003 found that tumors grew faster in men with low testosterone. Their cancer was more aggressive and those patients died sooner. [6]

At Harvard Medical School in 1996, eight doctors reported that "a high prevalence of biopsy-detectable prostate cancer was identified in men with low total or free testosterone." [7]

At the Memphis Veterans Administration Hospital in 1989, a group of nine researchers conducted a review of previous studies, concluding that elderly veterans lived longer when their testosterone levels were higher. They referred to studies as early as 1971. The higher the testosterone levels the longer the men lived. [8]

In an impressive collective effort between six international clinics, including UCLA and Columbia University in 1997, scientists used the Norwegian Cancer Registry to study the frozen blood serum and medical records of approximately 28,000 men. They found that healthy men actually had higher testosterone levels than the ones who developed prostate cancer. They concluded that the idea of testosterone increases the risk of prostate cancer is unsupported. This study is the second largest ever conducted on testosterone and prostate cancer. It is almost beyond belief that mainstream medicine should ignore conclusions based on 28,000 men. [9]

At the University of Chicago in 1991, a group of researchers concluded: "A separate analysis of serum testosterone levels revealed that the higher the pre-treatment serum testosterone level, the greater the survival rate. The higher the testosterone levels were, the longer the men lived and the better they fared. Doctors should be giving men testosterone therapy, rather than androgen ablation." [10]

At the University of Utah in 1997, thirteen researchers compared 214 sets of male twins. Men with higher testosterone levels had smaller prostate glands. [11]

At Tenovus Institute in Wales in 1984, over two hundred prostate cancer patients were studied. The men with the lowest testosterone levels had the poorest prognosis and died the soonest. The researchers concluded that "low concentrations of testosterone in plasma at the time of diagnosis related to a poor prognosis."[12]

At the Granada Medical Facility in 1978, eighteen men with BPH were studied and compared with healthy men of the same age group. Men with BPH had a 43% lower testosterone level than the healthy men. The men with BPH had an average level of only 2.3 ng/ml, while the levels averaged 4.0 ng/ml in healthy men. [13]

At the Royal London Hospital in 2000, nineteen doctors conducted a comprehensive review of thirty-four studies, concluding, "There has so far been no conclusive evidence, despite thirty-four studies, that levels of circulating testosterone in individuals developing prostate cancer are higher than in controls." [14]

At the Beth Israel Hospital in New York City in 1982, twenty-one researchers studied men for thirteen different hormones (or their metabolites) to determine which ones contributed to the growth of prostate cancer. The average cancer patient had a low testosterone level of about 350 ng/dl compared to the healthy men with levels averaging 450 ng/dl. In the men under sixty-five, the difference was much more dramatic, with levels of 282 ng in cancer patients compared to 434 ng for the healthy controls—over 50% higher testosterone in healthy men without cancer.[15]

At the internationally renowned Karolinska Institute in Sweden in 1996, a group of twenty-two researchers studied 2,400 cancer patients and found that the prostate cancer patients had 8% lower testosterone than healthy controls. The scientists concluded: "Testosterone levels were lower in patients with cancer than in controls."[16]

At the University of Utah in 1985, a large group of researchers studied the brothers of men with prostate cancer and found they had four times the chance of also getting cancer. The study showed that the high-risk brothers had much lower testosterone levels than healthy controls. [17]

At the University of Helsinki in 1983, twenty-four hormones were measured in men with BPH or prostate cancer, against healthy controls. The researchers in this study could not accept their own evidence, which showed that excess estrogens cause prostate disease, while high, youthful testosterone levels prevent it.[18]

At Boston University in 1954, twenty-five doctors studied men who were on testosterone therapy to see what effect it had on their prostate glands. These subjects had used testosterone propionate for four years. Healthy controls of the same age were compared. The men who were on testosterone therapy had less palpable irregularities and less hypertrophy than the healthy controls. Even using the wrong kind of testosterone resulted in better prostate health, fewer irregularities, and less BPH. Actually, they found less prostate disease of all kinds in testosterone-supplemented men.[19]

At the National Public Health Institute in Finland in 1999, a large cohort study on 62,440 Finnish men concluded, "The results of the current study do not appear to corroborate the hypothesis." that high levels of testosterone are linked to prostate disease. This is the largest study on record. [20]

At the International Agency for Research on Cancer, in France in 2000, a large group of researchers conducted a comprehensive review of the literature. Twenty-two major studies from around the world were analyzed. They reported, "The first conclusion of this review is that taken together, epidemiological studies have provided little support for the hypothesis that prostate cancer risk is increased in men with elevated total or bio-available testosterone." [21]

At Umea University Hospital in Sweden in 2003, almost 3,000 men both with and without prostate cancer were studied for androgen levels. The men with the highest levels of testosterone had the lowest rates of cancer, while the men with the lowest levels of testosterone had the highest rates of cancer. The doctors were stunned with the results because they began with a bias against testosterone and found that they had to reverse their hypothesis due to their own findings. [22]

It is always risky to challenge mainstream medical dogma. Many Doctors have lost their jobs for doing just that. In 2003, doctors at Harvard were not deterred from going against the prevailing negative view of testosterone and prostate health. They studied seventy-five men with low testosterone, twenty of whom had a pre-cancerous condition called "prostatic intraepithelial neoplasia," or PIN. They gave all of these men supplemental testosterone for one year knowing that the prevailing medical opinion was that the twenty men with PIN should be expected to get outright cancer of the prostate. Unsurprisingly, nothing of the sort happened. The men were in much better mental and physical health after raising their testosterone levels to normal ones, and their prostate glands prospered having the testosterone they needed. [23]

In 1981 at the University of Helsinki in Finland, a large group of researchers studied the hormone profiles of men with prostate cancer. The men who lived longest had a full 33% higher testosterone (T) level and a 67% higher progesterone level. The men who died the earliest had 33% higher estradiol and 36% higher estrone (several naturally occurring forms of estrogens. The researchers concluded, "In patients with a good response, the mean plasma testosterone level was significantly higher than in patients with poor response." [24]

Again at Helsinki University in Finland but in 1988, one hundred and twenty-three men (average age of seventy-two) with prostate cancer were studied for their hormone levels. The researchers concluded, "Low pre-treatment values (of testosterone) indicated poorer prognosis." A lower the free testosterone level was associated with a higher Gleason score. The lower the free testosterone the more aggressive and faster-growing the tumors. A lower free testosterone was associated with cancer metastasis. After four years, 80% of the men with the higher testosterone levels were still alive, but only 45 percent of the men with the lower testosterone levels were still alive. [25]

At the University of North Carolina in 1987, thirty-seven healthy men were compared to men with prostate cancer. The healthy men had 22% higher testosterone levels. [26]

At the University of Iowa in 1998, thirty-eight healthy men were injected with completely high levels of testosterone salts up to 500 mg weekly. "No significant change occurred in the prostate volume or serum PSA levels at any dose of exogenous testosterone." [27]

At the University of Iowa in 1996, thirty-nine men were injected with high levels of testosterone salts up to 500 mg. The concluded, however, that "Serum PSA is not responsive to elevated serum testosterone levels." [28]

At the Hamburg University Clinic in Germany in 1979, forty men were studied for hormone levels. The healthy men had higher testosterone levels, while the men with BPH and cancer had lower levels. [29]

At Harvard Medical School in 1995, forty-one researchers found that men with BPH had lower testosterone and androstenedione levels than healthy men and that estrogen dominance as men aged was a clear cause of hypertrophy.[30]

At Walter Reed Army Medical Center in Washington in 1995, forty-two hypogonadal men were administered either testosterone enanthate injections or transdermal testosterone. The researchers concluded, "This study suggests that in hypogonadal men neither PSMA [membrane antigen] nor PSA expression is testosterone-dependent." In other words, testosterone did not increase the risk of prostate cancer. [31]

At Adis International Ltd, in New Zealand in 1998, forty-five researchers gave transdermal testosterone to hypogonadal men for a year. As a result, their testosterone-to-estrogen ratios normalized and they experienced an improved erectile response, thereby improving their overall sexual function better. "PSA levels and prostate volumes remained in the normal range during long-term treatment." Supplementing testosterone improved sexual function and produced zero increased risk of prostate cancer. [32]

At Queen's University in Canada in 2002, a comprehensive review of the literature revealed: "The current evidence does not support the view that appropriate treatment of elderly hypogonadal men with androgens has a causal relationship with prostate cancer." [33]

At the Institute of Reproductive Medicine in Germany in 1999, forty-seven men were treated with transdermal testosterone for up to 10 years, and "prostate-specific antigen levels were constantly low in all patients." This long-term study showed no increased risk of prostate cancer.[34]

At the University of California at Los Angeles in 1995, forty-eight groups of men of diverse ethnic and racial background, averaging seventy years of age were studied. The Asian men with the highest levels of free testosterone had the lowest rates of prostate disease. Caucasians with the lowest levels of free testosterone had the highest rates of prostate disease.[35]

At the Imperial Cancer Research Fund in London in 1971, forty-nine men were studied for hormone levels. The healthy men had higher plasma testosterone levels than the men with prostate cancer and much higher levels than the men with advanced metastatic cancer.[36]

At the University of Medical Science in mainland China in 1993, fifty Chinese men were studied for serum testosterone levels. The healthy men had higher levels than the BPH or cancer patients.[37]

At the University of California at Davis in 1998, researchers reported on 51 patients indicating, "Men with prostate carcinoma and low testosterone levels have a much worse prognosis". [38]

At Nijmegen University Hospital in the Netherlands in 1990, a large group of researchers reported, "Low testosterone concentration at the start of therapy was also associated with poor prognosis."[39]

At Johns Hopkins University in 1993, fifty-three men with prostate cancer had decidedly lower DHEA and DHEA-S levels than healthy controls. [40]

At the Academy of Medicine in Poland in 1984, fifty-four men with BPH had lower levels of testosterone than the healthy controls. [41]

At the Veterans' Administration Centre in Los Angeles in 1968, a large group of physicians admitted that they saw no benefit from androgen ablation, even if the testosterone was lowered to zero. [42]

At the American Health Foundation in New York in 1982, fifty-six black men with prostate cancer were compared to healthy black men. The cancer patients had lower testosterone, androstenedione, and DHEA, while they also had higher estrone and estradiol levels.[43]

A study conducted at the University of Copenhagen over five years and consisting of two hundred forty-five men with prostate cancer showed that men with the highest levels of testosterone lived the longest by far with the highest quality-of-life and slowest growth of cancer. The men with the lowest levels died sooner and had a much lower quality-of-life with faster-growing malignancies. "Pretreatment level of serum testosterone was confirmed as having significant prognostic value on progression-free, overall and cancer-specific survival."[43]

German doctors in 2002 injected testosterone salts into 59 hypogonadal men over a period of three years. The prostate volume did not increase, the PSA did not rise, and there was no increase in rates of prostate disease of any kind.[45]

At the University of California in Torrance in 2003, sixty doctors gave natural testosterone transdermal gel to hypogonadal men for three years. The men received dramatic benefits, and "levels of PSA remained in the normal range."[46]

At the University of Utah in 1997, a research group of sixty-one doctors gave hypogonadal men injections and transdermal patches of testosterone, concluding, "Prostate size during therapy was comparable to that reported for normal men. In these men treated with transdermal testosterone, PSA levels were also within the normal range."[47]

At the University of Iowa in 1989, one hundred and ten men with prostate cancer were studied for testosterone levels. The higher the testosterone levels the slower the tumor growth and the longer they lived. "Patients with a pre-treatment testosterone level of fewer than 300 ng/100 ml ... had the most rapid progression."[48]

In 1977, doctors at the National Cancer Institute compared healthy men to those suffering from BPH. The healthy men had an average testosterone level 146% higher than the affected men. Once again running counter to the view of the medical establishment that high testosterone exacerbated or caused prostate cancer [49]

At the Roswell Institute in NY in 1980, sixty-four healthy men were compared to those with BPH. The healthy men had 152% more testosterone on the average than the patients.[50]

At the University of Tennessee in 1989, researchers conducted a study considering the longevity of men with prostate cancer. Higher testosterone was "the most significant variable" of all parameters studied in the longest-lived patients.[51]

At Beth Israel Center in 2004, a literature review of seventy-two studies showed that there was "no causal relationship between testosterone and prostate cancer risk."[52]

At the Cross Cancer Institute in Canada in 1991, men with the lowest testosterone levels died the soonest, and these men demonstrated also the highest rate of cancer growth.[53]

From 1999-2004, The National Health and Nutritional Examination Survey compared data from a study on age-related variations in the testosterone levels of 355 black and 631 white males. The results showed testosterone levels in black males decreased as they aged far more dramatically than white males. This may contribute to racial differences in prostate cancer.[54]

A retrospective review was conducted by the Department of Urology, Columbia University Medical Center, New York on 498 men in which they were evaluated for erectile dysfunction between January 2013 and July 2014. The study showed that men with erectile dysfunction and an elevated Body Mass Index, advanced age, or infrequent sexual activity appear to be at high risk of testosterone dysfunction.[55]

The Department of Pathology at the Federal Medical Centre, Idi-Aba, Abeokuta, Nigeria reported prostate cancer data on men of African descent, along with the carcinoma of the prostate and the cancer genome from men of African descent worldwide. The data found that men of African descent living in the USA and the Caribbean had the highest prostate cancer incidences. However, in Saharan African Men, tumor stage and grade were the highest.[56]

The Division of Urology at Beth Israel Deaconess Medical Center and Harvard Medical School together studied 117 patients who had been diagnosed with prostate cancer and treated by one physician between 1994 and 1997. After reviewing the clinical records, the researchers concluded that "patients with low versus normal free testosterone experienced an increased mean percentage of biopsies that showed cancer".[57]

In 2014, The Journal European Urology, conducted a literature review on the effects of serum testosterone on prostate cancer. According to their analysis, "high endogenous serum testosterone does not increase the risk of developing prostate cancer and low serum testosterone does not protect against prostate cancer." [58]

Department of Epidemiology, Harvard T.H. Chan School of Public Health conducted a case-control study that took place with 200 prostate cancer patients and 1057 controls from the Physicians' Health Study and Health Professionals Follow-up Study. They examined associations between pre-diagnostic circulating levels of total testosterone, free testosterone, DHT, androstanediol glucuronide, estradiol, and SHBG and risk of prostate cancer. The results showed that there may be some evidence that pre-diagnostic testosterone levels may be linked to prostate cancer.[59]

The New England Journal of Medicine conducted a one-year trial of seven hundred and ninety men, age 65 years old or older who were assigned serum testosterone concentration levels of less than 275 ng per deciliter. Men with symptoms of hypoandrogenism were given either testosterone gel or placebo gel for one year. The results showed that "in men 65 years of age or older, raising testosterone concentrations for one year from moderately low to the mid-normal range for men 19 to 40 years of age, had a moderate benefit with respect to sexual function and some benefit with respect to mood and depressive symptoms but no benefit with respect to vitality or walking distance".[60]

END NOTES

1. Prehn, Richmond T, On the Prevention and Therapy of Prostate Cancer by Androgen Administration. CANCER RESEARCH 59, 1 Sept. 1999, p 4161–4164., cancerres.aacrjournals. org/content/canres/59/17/4161.full.pdf.

2. Ribeiro, Maria M. Med.; Ruff, Paul M. Med.; Falkson, Geoffrey M. Med., M.D. Low Serum Testosterone and a Younger Age Predict for a Poor Outcome in Metastatic Prostate Cancer American Journal of Clinical Oncology: December 1997 - Volume 20 - Issue 6 - p 605-608, https://journals.lww.com/amjclinicaloncology/Abstract/1997/12000/Low_Serum_Testosterone_and_a_Younger_Age_Predict.15.aspx

3. Hubei Yike Daxue Xuebao 19 (1998), pp. 241-42 (NETA)

4. Georg Schatzl-Werner Reiter-Thomas Thürridl-Julia Waldmüller-Michael Roden-Stefan Söregi-Stephan Madersbacher. Endocrine Patterns in Patients with Benign and Malignant Prostatic Diseases - The Prostate - 2000 https://www.ncbi.nlm.nih.gov/pubmed/10906738

5. Schatzl G, Madersbacher S, Thurridl T, Waldmüller J, Kramer G, Haitel A, Marberger M. High-grade prostate cancer is associated with low serum testosterone levels. The Prostate. 2001 Apr 1;47(1):52-8.

6. Schatzl G, Madersbacher S, Haitel A, Gsur A, Preyer M, Haidinger G, Gassner C, Ochsner M, Marberger M. Associations of serum testosterone with microvessel density, androgen receptor density and androgen receptor gene polymorphism in prostate cancer. The Journal of urology. 2003 Apr 1;169(4):1312-5.

7. Morgentaler A, Bruning CO, Dewolf WC. Occult prostate cancer in men with low serum testosterone levels. Jama. 1996 Dec 18;276(23):1904-6.

8. Ishikawa S, Soloway MS, Van Der Zwaag R, Todd B. Prognostic factors in survival free of progression after androgen deprivation therapy for treatment of prostate cancer. The Journal of urology. 1989 May 1;141(5):1139-42.

9. Krieg M, Nass R, Tunn S. Effect of aging on endogenous level of 5 alpha-dihydrotestosterone, testosterone, estradiol, and estrone in epithelium and stroma of normal and hyperplastic human prostate. The Journal of Clinical Endocrinology & Metabolism. 1993 Aug 1;77(2):375-81.

10. Chodak GW, Vogelzang NJ, Caplan RJ, Soloway M, Smith JA. Independent Prognostic Factors in Patients With Metastatic (Stage D2) Prostate Cancer. JAMA. 1991;265(5):618–621. https://jamanetwork.com/journals/jama/article-abstract/384904

11. A. Wayne Meikle, Robert A. Stephenson, Cathryn M. Lewis, Richard G. Middleton. Effects of Age and Sex Hormones on Transition and Peripheral Zone Volumes of Prostate and Benign Prostatic Hyperplasia in Twins, The Journal of Clinical Endocrinology & Metabolism, Volume 82, Issue 2, 1 February 1997, P 571–575, https://doi.org/10.1210/jcem.82.2.3720

12. E Harper, M & G Pierrepoint, C & Griffiths, K. Carcinoma of the prostate: Relationship of pretreatment hormone levels to survival. European journal of cancer & clinical oncology. (1984). 20. 477-82. https://www.researchgate.net/publication/16769272_Carcinoma_of_the_prostate_Relationship_of_pretreatment_hormone_levels_to_survival

13. Ortega E, Ruiz E, Mendoza MC, Martin-Andres A. Plasma steroid and protein hormone concentrations in patients with benign prostatic hypertrophy and in normal men. Experientia. 1979 Jun 1;35(6):844-5.

14. Slater S, Oliver RT. Testosterone. Drugs & aging. 2000 Dec 1;17(6):431-9.

15. Zumoff B, Levin J, Strain GW, Rosenfeld RS, O'Connor J, Freed SZ, Kream J, Whitmore WS, Fukushima DK, Hellman L. Abnormal levels of plasma hormones in men with prostate cancer: Evidence toward a "two-disease" theory. The Prostate. 1982;3(6):579-88.

16. Gustafsson O, Norming U, Gustafsson S, Eneroth P, Åström G, Nyman CR. Dihydrotestosterone and testosterone levels in men screened for prostate cancer: a study of a randomized population. British journal of urology. 1996 Mar;77(3):433-40.

17. A. Wayne Meikle, William M. Stanish. Familial Prostatic Cancer Risk and Low Testosterone, The Journal of Clinical Endocrinology & Metabolism, Volume 54, Issue 6, 1 June 1982, p 1104–1108, https://doi.org/10.1210/jcem-54-6-1104

18. Sakari Rannikko, Herman Adlercreutz. Plasma estradiol, free testosterone, sex hormone binding globulin binding capacity, and prolactin in benign prostatic hyperplasia and prostatic cancer, Prostate 4 (1983), p. 223-29, https://doi.org/10.1002/pros.2990040302

19. Maurice A. Lesser, Samuel N. Vose, Grant M. Dixey. Effect Of Testosterone Propionate On The Prostate Gland Of Patients Over 45, ; The Journal of Clinical Endocrinology & Metabolism,

Volume 15, Issue 3, 1 March 1955, P 297–300, https://doi.org/10.1210/jcem-15-3-297

20. Ritva Heikkilä Ph.D. Kimmo Aho Ph.D. Markku Heliövaara M.D. Matti Hakama Sc.D. Jukka Marniemi Ph.D. Antti Reunanen M.D. Paul Knekt Ph.D. Serum testosterone and sex hormone-binding globulin concentrations and the risk of prostate carcinoma, Cancer Volume 86, Issue2 1999 p 312-315 https://onlinelibrary.wiley.com/doi/full/10.1002/%28SICI%291097-0142%2819990715%2986%3A2%3C312%3A%3AAID-CNCR15%3E3.0.CO%3B2-7

21. Kaaks R, Lukanova A, Sommersberg B. Plasma androgens, IGF-1, body size, and prostate cancer risk: a synthetic review. Prostate cancer and prostatic diseases. 2000 Nov;3(3):157.

22. Stattin, P., Lumme, S., Tenkanen, L., Alfthan, H., Jellum, E., Hallmans, G., Thoresen, S., Hakulinen, T., Luostarinen, T., Lehtinen, M., Dillner, J., Stenman, U. and Hakama, M. Int. J. High levels of circulating testosterone are not associated with increased prostate cancer risk: A pooled prospective study. Cancer, (2004) 108: p 418-424.https://onlinelibrary.wiley.com/doi/abs/10.1002/ijc.11572

23. Rhoden EL, Morgentaler A. Testosterone replacement therapy in hypogonadal men at high risk for prostate cancer: Results of 1 year of treatment in men with prostatic intraepithelial neoplasia. J Urol. 2003;170:2348–51. https://www.ncbi.nlm.nih.gov/pubmed/14634413

24. Adlercreutz H, Rannikko S, Kairento AL, Karonen SL. Hormonal pattern in prostatic cancer. Acta endocrinologica. 1981 Dec 1;98(4):634-40.

25. Haapiainen R, Rannikko S, Alfthan O, Adlercreutz H. Pretreatment plasma levels of testosterone and sex hormone binding globulin binding capacity in relation to clinical staging and survival in prostatic cancer patients. The prostate. 1988;12(4):325-32.26. J. Clin. Endoc. Metab. 77 (1993) pp. 375-81

26. Hulka BS, Checkoway H, Hammond JE, Ferdinando GD, Mickey DD, Fried FA, Stumpf WE, Beckman Jr WC, Clark TD. Serum hormone levels among patients with prostatic carcinoma or benign prostatic hyperplasia and clinic controls. The Prostate. 1987;11(2):171-82.

27. Cooper CS, MacIndoe JH, Perry PJ, Yates WR, Williams RD. The effect of exogenous testosterone on total and free prostate specific antigen levels in healthy young men. The Journal of urology. 1996 Aug 1;156(2):438-42.

28. Cooper CS, Perry PJ, Sparks AE, MacIndoe JH, Yates WR, Williams RD. Effect of exogenous testosterone on prostate volume, serum and semen prostate specific antigen levels in healthy young men. The Journal of urology. 1998 Feb 1;159(2):441-3.29. J. Urol 156 (1996) pp. 438-42

29. Acta Endocrinologica 90 (1979), pp. 77-36

30. Gann PH, Hennekens CH, Grodstein F, Stampfer MJ, Longcope C, Verhoek-Oftedahl W. A prospective study of plasma hormone levels, nonhormonal factors, and development of benign prostatic hyperplasia. The prostate. 1995 Jan;26(1):40-9.

31. Douglas TH, Connelly RR, McLeod DG, Erickson SJ, Iii RB, Murphy GP. Effect of exogenous testosterone replacement on prostate-specific antigen and prostate-specific membrane antigen levels in hypogonadal men. Journal of surgical oncology. 1995 Aug;59(4):246-50.

32. McClellan KJ, Goa KL. Transdermal testosterone. Drugs. 1998 Feb 1;55(2):253-8.

33. Morales A. Androgen replacement therapy and prostate safety. European urology. 2002 Feb 1;41(2):113-20.

34. Behre HM, Von Eckardstein S, Kliesch S, Nieschlag E. Long-term substitution therapy of hypogonadal men with transscrotal testosterone over 7–10 years. Clinical Endocrinology. 1999 May;50(5):629-35.36. Cancer Epidimiology Biomarkers & Preview 4 (1995), pp.735-41

35. Wu AH, Whittemore AS, Kolonel LN, John EM, Gallagher RP, West DW, Hankin J, Teh CZ, Dreon DM, Paffenbarger RS. Serum androgens and sex hormone-binding globulins in relation to lifestyle factors in older African-American, white, and Asian men in the United States and Canada. Cancer Epidemiology and Prevention Biomarkers. 1995 Oct 1;4(7):735-41.

36. British Journal of Medicine 4 (1971), pp. 391-94

37. Hejishu 16 (1993), pp. 649-52

38. Daniell HW. A worse prognosis for men with testicular atrophy at therapeutic orchiectomy

for prostate carcinoma. Cancer: Interdisciplinary International Journal of the American Cancer Society. 1998 Sep 15;83(6):1170-3.

39. Mulders PF, Dijkman GA, Moral PF, Theeuwes AG, Debruyne FM. Analysis of prognostic factors in disseminated prostatic cancer. An update. Cancer. 1990 Jun 15;65(12):2758-61. 41. Cancer Epidemiology Biomarkers & Preven. 2 (1993), pp. 219-21

40. Comstock GW, Gordon GB, Hsing AW. The relationship of serum dehydroepiandrosterone and its sulfate to subsequent cancer of the prostate. Cancer Epidemiology and Prevention Biomarkers. 1993 May 1;2(3):219-21.

41. Akad. Med. Bialymstoku Supp. 42 (1984), p. 17

42. Young HH, Kent JR. Plasma testosterone levels in patients with prostatic carcinoma before and after treatment. The Journal of urology. 1968 Jun 1;99(6):788-92.

43. Hill P, Wynder EL, Garbaczewski L, Walker AR. Effect of diet on plasma and urinary hormones in South African black men with prostatic cancer. Cancer research. 1982 Sep 1;42(9):3864-9.

44. Iversen P, Rasmussen F, Christensen IJ. Serum testosterone as a prognostic factor in patients with advanced prostatic carcinoma. Scandinavian journal of urology and nephrology. Supplementum. 1994;157:41-7.

45. Von Eckardstein S, Nieschlag E. Treatment of male hypogonadism with testosterone undecanoate injected at extended intervals of 12 weeks: a phase II study. Journal of andrology. 2002 May 6;23(3):419-25.

46. Swerdloff RS, Wang C. Three-year follow-up of androgen treatment in hypogonadal men: preliminary report with testosterone gel. The Aging Male. 2003 Jan 1;6(3):207-11.

47. Meikle AW, Arver S, Dobs AS, Adolfsson J, Sanders SW, Middleton RG, Stephenson RA, Hoover DR, Rajaram L, Mazer NA. Prostate size in hypogonadal men treated with a nonscrotal permeation-enhanced testosterone transdermal system. Urology. 1997 Feb 1;49(2):191-6.

48. Ishikawa S, Soloway MS, Van Der Zwaag R, Todd B. Prognostic factors in survival free of progression after androgen deprivation therapy for treatment of prostate cancer. The Journal of urology. 1989 May 1;141(5):1139-42.

49. Saroff J, Kirdani RY, Chu M, Wajsman Z, Murphy GP. Measurements of prolactin and androgens in patients with prostatic diseases. Oncology. 1980;37(1):46-52.

50. Saroff J, Kirdani RY, Chu M, Wajsman Z, Murphy GP. Measurements of prolactin and androgens in patients with prostatic diseases. Oncology. 1980;37(1):46-52.

51. Soloway MS, Ishikawa S, Van Der Zwaag R, Todd B. Prognostic factors in patients with advanced prostate cancer. Urology. 1989 May 1;33(5):53-6.

52. Rhoden EL, Morgentaler A. Risks of testosterone-replacement therapy and recommendations for monitoring. New England Journal of Medicine. 2004 Jan 29;350(5):482-92.

53. Ernst DS, Hanson J, Venner PM. Analysis of prognostic factors in men with metastatic prostate cancer. The Journal of urology. 1991 Aug 1;146(2):372-6.

54. Hu H, Odedina FT, Reams RR, Lissaker CT, Xu X. Racial differences in age-related variations of testosterone levels among US males: Potential implications for prostate cancer and personalized medication. Journal of racial and ethnic health disparities. 2015 Mar 1;2(1):69-76.

55. Pagano MJ, De Fazio A, Levy A, RoyChoudhury A, Stahl PJ. Age, body mass index, and frequency of sexual activity are independent predictors of testosterone deficiency in men with erectile dysfunction. Urology. 2016 Apr 1;90:112-8.

56. Rebbeck TR, Devesa SS, Chang BL, Bunker CH, Cheng I, Cooney K, Eeles R, Fernandez P, Giri VN, Gueye SM, Haiman CA. Global patterns of prostate cancer incidence, aggressiveness, and mortality in men of african descent. Prostate cancer. 2013;2013.

57. Hoffman MA, DeWOLF WC, Morgentaler A. Is low serum free testosterone a marker for high grade prostate cancer?. The Journal of urology. 2000 Mar 1;163(3):824-7.

58. Khera M, Morgentaler, A. Reply To Julia Klap And Kevin R. Loughlin's Letter To The Editor Re: Mohit Khera, David Crawford, Alvaro Morales, Andrea Salonia, Abraham Morgentaler. A New Era Of Testosterone And Prostate Cancer: From Physiology To Clinical Implications. European urology. 2014 (65):115-23.

59. Graff RE, Meisner A, Ahearn TU, Fiorentino M, Loda M, Giovannucci EL, Mucci LA, Pettersson A. Pre-diagnostic circulating sex hormone levels and risk of prostate cancer by ERG tumour protein expression. British Journal of Cancer. 2016 Apr;114(8):939.

60. Seftel AD. Re: Effects of Testosterone Treatment in Older Men. The Journal of urology. 2016 Aug 1;196(2):516-9.

REFERENCES

Abrams, D. I. An integrative approach to prostate cancer. *The Journal of Alternative and Complementary Medicine*. 2018;24(9-10):872-880. https://doi.org/10.1089/acm.2018.0169

Advea, M. M., Souto, G. Diet-induced metabolic acidosis. *Clinical Nutrition*. 2011;30:416-421. https://doi.org/10.1016/j.clnu.2011.03.008

Alcaraz, A. Hammerer, P., Tubaro, A., Schröder, F. H., Castro, R. Is there evidence of a relationship between benign prostatic hyperplasia and prostate cancer: Findings of a literature review. *European Urology*. 2009;55:864-875. https://doi.org.10.1016/j.eururo.2008.11.011

American Cancer Society. "Estimated Number of New Cancer Cases and Deaths by Sex, US, 2018." *American Cancer Society: Cancer Facts & Figures 2018*. https://www.cancer.org/research/cancer-facts-statistics/all-cancer-facts-figures/cancer-facts-figures-2018.html

Ahn, A. C., Tewari, M., Poon, C., Phillips, R. S. The limits of reductionism in medicine: Could systems biology offer an alternative? *PLoS Medicine*. 2006; 3(6):e208. https://doi.org/10.1371/journal.pmed.0030208

Ahn, A. C., Tewari, M., Poon, C., Phillips, R. S. The clinical applications of a systems approach. PLoS Medicine. 2006;3(6):e209. https://doi.org/10.1371/journal.pmed.0030209.g001

Berges, R. R., Kassen, A., Senge, T. Treatment of symptomatic benign prostatic hyperplasia with Beta-sitosterol: An 18-month follow-up. *BJU International*. 2000;85(7):842-846.

Berges, R. R., Windeler, J., Trampisch, H. J., Senge, T. Randomised, placebo-controlled, double-blind clinical trial of Beta-sitosterol in patients with benign prostatic hyperplasia. Beta-sitosterol Study Group. *Lancet*. 1995;345(8964)1529-1532.

Bernstein, A. N., Shoag, J. E., Golan, R., Halpern, J. A., Schaeffer, E. M., Hsu, W. Nguyen, P. L., Sedrakyan, A., Chen, R. C., Eggener, S., E., Hu, J., C. Contemporary incidence and outcomes of prostate cancer lymph node metastases. *Journal of Urology*. 2018;199:1510-1517. https://doi.org.10.1016/j.juro.2017.12.048

Bostanci, Y., Kazzazi, A., Momtahen, S., Laze, J., Djavan, B. Correlation between benign prostatic hyperplasia and inflammation. *Current Opinions in Urology*. 2013;23(1):5-10. https://doi.org/10.1097/MOU.0b013e32835abd4a

Bostwick, D. G., Cooner, W. H., Denis, L., Jones, G. W., Scardino, P. T., Murphy, G. P. The association of benign prostatic hyperplasia and cancer of the prostate. *Cancer Supplement*. 1992;70:291-301.

Boyle, P., Robertson, C., Mazzetta, C., Keech, M., Hobbs, R., Fourcade, R., Kiemeney, L., Lee, C., The association between lower urinary tract symptoms and erectile dysfunction in four centres: The UrEpik study. *BJU International*. 2003;92(7):719-725. https://doi.org/10.1046/j.1464-410X.2003.04449.x

Bowers, J. How much sugar is in popular drinks? *The Diabetes Council*. https://www.thediabetescouncil.com/how-much-sugar-is-in-popular-drinks/

Braun, M. H., Sommer, F., Haupt, G., Mathers, M. J., Reifenrath, B., Engelmann, U. H. Lower urinary tract symptoms and erectile dysfunction: Co-morbidity or typical "Aging Male" symptoms? Results of the "Cologne Male Survey." *European Urology*. 2003;44(5):588-594. https://doi.org/10.106/SO302-2838(03)00358-0

Bray, G. A. Energy and fructose from beverages sweetened with sugar or high-fructose corn syrup pose a health risk for some people. *Advanced Nutrition*. 2013;4:220-225. https://doi.org/10.3945/an.112002816

Bray, G. A. How bad is fructose? *American Journal of Clinical Nutrition*. 2007;86:895-896.

Cavarretta, I., Mancini, N., Salonia, A. Analysis of the enteric microbiome: First tentative steps towards a comprehensive work-up of prostate cancer? *European Urology*. 2018:583-584. https://doi.org/10.1016/j.eururo.2018.07.009

Chambliss, W. G. A critical review of Graminex flower pollen extract for symptomatic relieve of lower urinary tract symptoms (LUTS) in men. *Flower Pollen Extract and its Effect for Prostate Health*. 2003:4-9.

Chasapis, C. T. Loutsidou, A. C., Spiliopoulou, C. A., Stefanidou, M. E. Zinc and human health: An update. *Archives in Toxicology*. 2012;86(4):521-534. https://doi.org/10.007/s00204-011-0775-1

Church, T. S., Thomas, D. M., Tudor-Locke, C., Katzmarzyk, P.T., Earnest, C. P., Rodarte, R. Q., Martin, C. K., Blair, S., N., Bouchard, C. Trends over 5 decades of U.S. occupation-related physical activity and their associations with obesity. *PloS One*. 2011;6(5):e19657. https://doi.org/10.1371/journal.pone.0019657

Coffey, D. S. Similarities of prostate and breast cancer: Evolution, diet, and estrogens. *Urology*. 2001;57(Suppl 4A):31-38.

Cohen, N. M., Tulsi – Ocimum sanctum: A herb for all reasons. Journal of Ayurveda *Integrative Medicine*. 2014;5(4):251-259. https://doi.org/10.4103/0975-9476.146554

Cordain, L., Eaton, S. B., Sebastian, A. Mann, N., Lindeberg, S., Watkins, B. A., O'Keefe, J. H, Brand-Miller, J. Origins and evolution of the Western diet: Health implications for the 21st century. *The*

American Journal of Clinical Nutrition. 2005;81(2):341-354. https://doi.org/10.1093/ajcn.81.2.341

Costello, L. C., Franklin, R. B. A comprehensive review of the role of zinc in normal prostate function and metabolism; and its implications in prostate cancer. *Archives in Biochemistry and Biophysiology.* 2016;611:100-112. https://doi.org/10.1016/j.abb2016.04.014

Daniel, C. R., Cross, A. J., Koebnick, C., Sinha, R. Trends in meat consumption in the United States. *Public Health Nutrition.* 2011; 14(4):575-583. https://doi.org/10.1017/S1368980010002077

Dairiki Shortliffe, L. M., Sellers, R. G., Schachter, J., The characterization of nonbacterial prostatitis: Search for an etiology. *The Journal of Urology.* 1992;148:1461-1466.

Davis, N. J., Vaughan, C. P., Johnson, T. M., Goode, P. S., Burgio, K. L., Redden, D. T., Markland, A. D. Caffeine intake and its association with urinary incontinence in United States Men: Results from National Health and Nutrition Examination Surveys 2005–2006 and 2007–2008. *Proceedings from the American Urological Association. Journal of Urology.* 2012;189(6)2170-2174. https://doi.org/10.1016/j.juro.2012.12.061

Delongchamps, N. B., de la Roza, G., Chandan, V., Jones, R., Sunheimer, R., Threatte, G., Jumbelic, M., Haas, G. P. Evaluation of prostatitis in autopsied prostates—Is chronic inflammation associated with benign prostatic hyperplasia or cancer? *Journal of Urology.* 2008;179(5):1736-1740. https://doi.org/10.1016/j.juro.2008.01.034

De Nunzi, C., Kramer, G., Marberger, M., Montironi, R., Nelson, W., Shröder, F., Sciarra, A., Tubaro, A. The controversial relationship between benign prostatic hyperplasia and prostate cancer: The role of inflammation. *European Urology.* 2011;60:106-117. https://doi.org.10.1016.j.eururo.2011.03.055

Duffey, K. J., Popkin, B. M. High-fructose corn syrup: Is this what's for dinner? *American Journal of Clinical Nutrition.* 2008;88(suppl):1722S-1732S. https://doi.org/10.3945/ajcn.2008.25825C

Eaton, S. B., Eaton III, S. B., Konner, M. J. Paleolithic nutrition revisited: A twelve-year retrospective on its nature and implications. *European Journal of Clinical Nutrition.* 1997;51:207-216.

Elkahwaji, J. E. The role of inflammatory mediators in the development of prostatic hyperplasia and prostate cancer. *Research and Reports in Urology.* 2013;5:1-10. https://dx.doi.org/10.2147.RRU.S23386

Fedorovich, S. V., Voronina, P. P., Waseem, T. V. Ketogenic diet versus ketoacidosis: What determines the influence of ketone bodies on neurons? *Neural Regeneration Research.* 2018;13(12):2060-2063. https://doi.org/10.4103/1673-5374.241442

Fields, S. The fat of the land: Do agricultural subsidies foster poor health? *Environmental Health Perspectives.* 2004;112(14):A21-A23. https://www.ncbi.nlm.nih.gov/pmc/articles/PMC1247588/pdf/ehp0112-a00820.pdf

Frassetto, L. A., Schloetter, M., Mietus-Synder, M., Morris, R. C., Sebastian, A. Metabolic and physiologic improvements from consuming a paleolithic, hunter-gather type diet. *European Journal of Clinical Nutrition.* 2009;63:947-955.

Frassetto, L., Morris, R. C. Jr., Sellmeyer, D. E., Todd, K., Sebastian, A., Diet, evolution and aging—the pathophysiologic effects of the post-agricultural inversion of the potassium-to-sodium and base-to-chloride ratios in the human diet. *European Journal of Nutrition.* 2001;40(5):200-213.

Fuller, F. China's growing market for dairy products. *Iowa Agricultural Review.* 2004;10(3)

Ganmaa, D., Li, X., Wang, J., Qin, L., Wang, P., Sato, A. Incidence and mortality of testicular and prostatic cancers in relation to world dietary practices. *International Journal of Cancer.* 2002;98:262-267.

Gasior, M., Rogawski, M. A., Hartman, A. L. Neuroprotective and disease-modifying effects of the ketogenic diet. *Behavioral Pharmacology.* 2006;17(5-6):431-439.

Gillis, C., N. Panax ginseng pharmacology: A nitric oxide link? *Biochemical pharmacology.* 1997;54(1):1-8. https://doi.org/10.1016/S0006-2952(97)00193-7

Grattan, B. J. Jr., Plant sterols as anticancer nutrients: Evidence for their role in breast cancer. *Nutrients.* 2013;5(2):359-387. https://doi.org/10.3390/nu5020359

Gustafsson, O., Norming, U., Gustafsson, S., Eneroth, P., Aström, G., Nymon, C.R. Dihydrotestosterone and testosterone levels in men screened for prostate cancer: A study of a randomized population. *British Journal of Urology.* 1996;77:433-440. https://doi.org/10.1046/j.1464-410X.1996.89120.x

Haapiainen, R, Rannikko, S., Alfthan, O., Adlercreutz, H. Pretreatment plasma levels of testosterone and sex hormone binding globulin binding capacity in relation to clinical staging and survival of prostatic cancer patients. *Prostate.* 1988;12:325-332. https://doi.org/10.1002/pros.2990120406.

Heikkilä, R., Aho, K., Heliövaara, M., Hakama, M., Marniemi, J., Reunanen, A., Knekt, P. Serum testosterone and sex hormone-binding globulin concerntations and the risk of prostate carcinoma: A longitudinal study. *Cancer.* 1999;86:312-315. https://doi.org/10.1002.(SICI)1097-1042(19990715)86:2<312::AID-CNCR15>3.0.CO;2-7

Henning, S. M., Wang, P., Carpenter, C. L., Heber, D. Epigenetic effects of green tea polyphenols in cancer. *Future Medicine.* 2013. https://doi.org/10.2217/epi.13.57

Jena, A. K., Vasisht, K., Sharma, N., Kaur, R., Dhingra, M. S., Karan, M. Amelioration of testosterone induced benign prostatic hyperplasia by Prunus species. *Journal of Ethnopharmacology.* 2016;190:33-45. https://doi.org/10.1016/j.jep.2016.05.052

Jothie, R. E., Illuri, R., Bethapudi, B., Anandhakumar, S., Bhaskar, A., Chinampudur, V. C., Munkinajeddu, D., Agarwal, A. Anti-stress activity in Ocimum sanctum: Possible effects of Hypothalamic-Pituitary-

Adrenal Axis. *Phytotherapy Research*. 2016;30(5):805-814. https://doi.org/10.1002/ptr.5584

Kaaks, R, Lukanova, A., Sommersberg, B. Plasma androgens, IGF-1, body size, and prostate cancer risk: A synthetic review. *Prostate Cancer and Prostatic Diseases*. 2000;3(3):157-172. https://doi.org/10.1038.sj.pcan.4500421

Kamenov, Z., Fileva, S., Kalinov, K., Jannini, E. A. Evaluation of the efficacy and safety of Tribulus terrestris in male sexual dysfunction – A prospective, randomized, double-blind, placebo-controlled clinical trial. *Maturitas*. 2017;99:20-26. https://doi.org/10.1016/j.maturitas.2017.01.011

Karsten, H. D., Patterson, P. H., Stout, R., Crews, G. Vitamins A, E and fatty acid composition of the eggs of caged hens and pastured hens. *Renewable Agriculture and Food Systems*. 2010;25(1):45-54. https://doi.org/10.1017/S1742170599990214

Khera, M., Crawford, D., Morales, A., Salonia, A., Morgentaler, A. A new era of testosterone and prostate cancer: From physiology to clinical implications. 2014; 65(1)115-223. https://doi.org/10.1016/j.eurouro.2013.08.015

Kim, S.W., Phytotherapy: Emerging therapeutic option in urologic disease. *Tranlational Andrology and Urology*. 2012;1(3):181-191. https://doi.org/10.3978/j.issn.2223-4683.2012.05.10

Kubatka, P., Kello, M., Kajo, K., Kruzliak, P., Výbohová, D., Mojžiš, J., et al. Oregano demonstrates distinct tumour-suppressive effects in the breast carcinoma model. *European Journal of Nutrition*. 2017;56(3):1303-1316. https://doi.org/10.1007/s00394-016-1181-5

Kurano, M., Hasegawa, K., Kunimi, M., Hara, M., Yatomi, Y., Teramoto, T., Tsukamoto, K. Sitosterol prevents obesity-related chronic inflammation. *BBA Molecular and Cell Biology of Lipids*. 2018;1863(2):191-198. https://doi.org/10.1016/j.bbalip.2017.12.004

Lambert, J. D., Elias, R. J. The antioxidant and pro-oxidant activities of green tea polyphenols: A role in cancer prevention. *Archives of Biochemistry and Biophysiology*. 2010;501(1):65-72. https://doi.org/10.1016/j.abb.2010.06.013

Lapointe, J., Li, C., Higgins, J. P., van de Rign, M., Bair, E., Montgomery, K., et al. Gene expression profiling identifies clinically relevant subtypes of prostate cancer. *Proceedings of the National Academy of Sciences of the United States*. 2004;101(3):811-816. https://doi.org/10.1073/pnas.0304146101

Lau, E., Cooper, C. The epidemiology of osteoporosis: The Oriental perspective in a world context. *Clinical orthopaedics and related research*. 1996;323:65-74.

LaVallee, R. A., Kim, T., Yi, H. Apparent per capita alcohol consumption: National, state, and regional trends, 1977-2012. *National Institute of Alcohol Abuse and Alcoholism*. 2014. U. S. Department of Health and Human Services. Public Health Service. National Institutes of Health. https://pubs.niaaa.nih.gov/publications/surveillance98/CONS12.htm

Leung, P., Aronson, W. J., Ngo, T. H., Golding, L. A., Barnard, R. J. Exercise alters the IGF axis in vivo and increases p53 protein in prostate tumor cells in vitro. *Journal of Applied Physiology*. 2004;96:450-454. https://doi.org/10.1152/japplphysiol.00871.2003

Leyva-López, N., Gutiérrez/Grijalva, E. P. Essential oils of oregano: Biological activity beyond their antimicrobial properties. *Molecules*. 2017;22(6):989. https://doi.org/10.3390/molecules22060989

Lindeberg, S., Cordain, L., Eaton, S. B. Biological and clinical potential of a paleolithic diet. *Journal of Nutritional & Environmental Medicine*. 2009;13(3):149-160. https://doi.org/10.1080/13590840310001619397

MacKay, D., J. Nutrients and botanicals for erectile dysfunction: Examining the evidence. *Alternative Medicine Review*. 2004;9(1):4-16.

Mann, N. J. Paleolithic nutrition: What can we learn from the past? *Asia Pacific Journal of Clinical Nutrition*. 2004;13Suppl:17.

Mengmeng, L., Xingya, Z., Wang, H., Wang, F., Guan, W. Roles of caloric restriction, ketogenic diet and intermittent fasting during initiation, progression and metastasis of cancer in animal models: A systemic review and meta-analysis. *PLoSone*. 2014. https://doi.org/10.1371/journal.pone.0115137

Morgentaler, A. Testosterone and prostate cancer: An historical perspective on a modern myth. *European Urology*. 2006;50(5):935-939. https://doi.org/10.1016/j.eururo.2006.06.034

Mulvey, L., Chandrasekaren, A., Liu, K., Lombardi, S., Wang, X. P., Auborn, K. J., Goodwin, L. Interplay of genes regulated by estrogen and diindolylmethane in breast cancer cell lines. *Molecular Medicine*. 2007;13(1-2):69-78. https://doi.org/10.2119/2006-00038.Mulvey

Nasri, H., Baradaran, A., Shirzad, H., Rafieian-Kopaei, M. New concepts in nutraceuticals as alternatives to pharmaceuticals. *Integrative Journal of Preventive Medicine*. 2014;5(12):1487-1499.

Nestle, M. *Food Politics: How the Food Industry Influences Nutrition and Health*. 2013. Berkeley, CA: University of California Press. 11-12.

Niedzwiecki, A., Roomi, M. V., Kalinovsky, T., Rath, M. Anticancer efficacy in polyphenols and their combinations. *Nutrients*. 2016;8(9):E552. https://doi.org/10.3390/nu8090552

Nocerino, E., Amato, M., Izzo, A. A. The aphrodisiac and adaptogenic properties of ginseng. *Fitoterapia*. 2000:S1-5.

Ogden, C. L., Yanovski, S. Z., Carroll, M. D., Flegal, K. M., The epidemiology of obesity. *Gastroenterology*. 2007;132(6):2087-2102. https://doi/org/10.1053/j.gastro.2007.03.052

O'Keefe, J. H., Cordain, L. Cardiovascular disease resulting from a diet and lifestyle at odds with our paleolithic genome: How to become a 21st-century hunter-gathering. *Mayo Clinic Proceedings*. 2004;79(1):101-108. https://doi.org/10.4065/79.1.101

Olvera-Caltzontzin, P. Delgado, G., Aceves, C., Anguiano, B., Iodine uptake in prostate cancer in the TRAMP mouse model. *Molecular Medicine*. 2013;19(1):409-416. https://doi.org/10.2119/molmed.2013.00093

Ornish, D., Weidner, G., Fair, W. R., Marlin, R., Pettengill, E. B., Raisin, C. J., et al. Intensive lifestyle changes may affect the progression of prostate cancer. *Journal of Urology*. 2005;174:1065-1070. https://doi.org/10.1097/01.ju.0000169487.49018.73

Palapattu, G. S., Sutcliffe, S., Bastian, P. J., Platz, E. A., De Marzo, A. M., Isaacs, W. B., Nelson, W. G. Prostate carcinogenesis and inflammation: Emerging insights. *Carcingoenesis*. 2005;26(7):1170-1181. https://doi.org/10.1093/carcin/bgh317

Paniagua-Pérez, R., Flores-Mondragón, G., Reyes-Legorreta, C. Herera-López, B., Cervantes-Hernández, I., Maddrigal-Santillán, O. Evaluation of the anti-inflammatory capacity of Beta-sitosterol in rodent assays. *African Journal of Complementary and Alternative Medicine*. 2016;14(1)123-130. https://doi.org/10.21010/ajtcam.v14i1.13

Pernar, C. H., Ebot, E. M., Pettersson, A., Graff, R. E., Giunchi, F., Aheam, T. U., et al. A prospective study of the association between physical activity and risk of prostate cancer defined by clinical features and TEMPRSS2:ERG. *European Urology*. 2018;S0302-2838(18)30730-30739. https://doi.org/10.1016/j.eurouro.2018.09.041

Pizzorno, J., Frassetto, L.A., Katzinger, J. Diet-induced acidosis: Is it real and clinically relevant? *British Journal of Nutrition*. (2010);103:1185-1194. https://doi/org/10.1017/S0007114509993047

Pizzorno, L., Nothing boring about boron. *Integrative Medicine (Encinitas)*. 2015;14(4):35-48.

Porter, C. M., Shrestha, E., Peiffer, L. B., Sfanos, K. S. The microbiome in prostate inflammation and prostate cancer. *Prostate Cancer and Prostatic Diseases*. 2018;21:345-354. https://doi.org/10.1028/s41391-018-0041-1

Potter, G. A., Burke, M. D. Salvestrols—Natural products with tumour selective activity. *Journal of Orthomolecular Medicine*. 2006;21(1):34-36.

Prakash, P., Gupta, N. Therapeutic uses of Ociumum sanctum linn (tulsi) with a note on eugenol and its pharmacological actions: A short review. *Indian Journal of Physiology and Pharmacology*. 2005;49(2):125-131.

Rahkovsky, I., Young, J., Carlson, A. Consumers balance time and money in purchasing convenience foods. *United States Department of Agriculture*. 2018. https://www.ers.usda.gov/webdocs/

publications/89344/err251_summary.pdf?v=0

Rangul, V., Sund, E. R., Mork, P. J., Røe, O., D., Bauman, A. The associations of sitting time and physical activity on total and site-specific cancer incidence: Results from the HUNT study, Norway. *PLoS One*. 2018; 13(10):e0206015. https://doi.org/10.1371/journal.pone.0206015

Rietjens, I. M. C. M., Louisse, J., Beekman, K. The potential effects of phytoestrogens. *British Journal of Pharmacology*. 2017;174(11):1263-1280. https://doi.org/10.1111/bph.13622

Roehrborn, C. G., Egan, K. B., Miner, N. M., Ni, X., Wong, D. G., Rosen, R. C. Erectile dysfunction and lower urinary tract symptoms associated with benign prostatic hyperplasia (LUTS/BPH) combined responders to tadalafil after 12 weeks of treatment. *BJU International*. 2016;118(1):153-160. https://doi.org//10.1111/bju.13406.Epub2016Feb11

Rosen, R., Altwein, J., Boyle, P., Kirby, R. S., Lukacs, B., Meuleman, E., O'Leary, M. P., Puppo, P. Robertson, C., Giuliano, F. Lower urinary tract symptoms and male sexual dysfunction: The multinational survey of the aging male (MSAM-7). *European Urology*. 2003:44(6):637-649. https://doi.org/10.1016/j.eururo.2003.08.015

Ross, R. K., Coetzee, G. A., Reichardt, J., Skinner, E., Henderson, B. E., Does the racial-ethnic variation in prostate cancer risk have a hormonal basis? *Cancer*. 1995;75:1778-1782. https://doi.org/10.1002/1097-0142(19950401)75:7+<1778::AID-CNR2820751605>3.0.CO;2-J

Rundqvist, H., Augsten, M., Strömberg, A., Rullman, R., Mijwel, S., Kharasiha, P., et al. Effect of acute exercise on prostate cancer cell growth. *PLosOne*. 2013. https://doi.org/10.1371/journal.pone.0067579

Sayeed, B., Ameen, S. S. Beta-Sitosterol: A promising but orphan nutraceutical to fight against cancer. *Nutrition and Cancer*. 2015:67(8)1214-1220. https://doi.org/10.1080/01635581.2015.1087042

Schaefer, B. A., Tan, H. L., Burke, M. D., Potter, G. A. Nutrition and cancer: Salvestrol case studies. *Journal of Orthomolecular Medicine*. 2007;22(4):177-182.

Sciarra, A., Di Silverio, F., Salciccia, S., Autran Gomez, A. M., Gentile, V. Inflammation and chronic prostatic diseases: Evidence for a link? *European Urology*. 2007;52(4):964-972. https://doi.org/10.1016/j.eururo.2007.06.038

Shenkin, A. The role of minerals and trace elements in relation to long-term health and chronic disease. In S. P. Allison and V. L. W. Go (eds). *Metabolic Issues of Clinical Nutrition*. Nestlé Nutrition Workshop Series Clinical & Performance Program, vol 9. (Basel: Nestec Ltd., Vevey/S. Karger AG).2004. pp 169-185.

Shindel, A. W., Zin, Z. C., Lin, G., Fandel, T. M., Huang, Y. C., Banie, L., Breyer, B. N., Garcia, N. M., Lin, C. S., Lue, T. F. Erectogenic and neurotrophic effects of icariin, a purified extract of horny goat weed

(Epimedium spp.) in vitro and in vivo. *Journal of Sexual Medicine.* 2010;7(4 Pt 1):1518-1528. https://doi.org/10.111/j.1743-6109.2009.01699.x

Simpson, R. J., Benign prostatic hyperplasia. *British Journal of General Practice.* 1997;47:235-240.

Soloway, M. S., Ishikawa, S., Van Der Zwaag, R., Todd, B., Prognostic factors in patients with advanced prostate cancer. *Urology.* 1999;33(5):53-56.
https://doi.org/10.1016/0090-4295(89)90107-6

Stasiak, M., Żarłok, K., Tomaszewski, W. Erectile dysfunction – Treatment with substances of natural origin. *Wiad Lek.* 2016;69(3 pt 2):576-581.

Stattin, P., Lumme S., Tenkanen, L., Alfthan, H., Jellum E., Hallmans, G., Thoresen, S., Hakulinen, T., Luostarinen, T., Lethinen, M., Dilner, J., Stenman, U. H., Hakama, M. High levels of circulating testosterone are not associated with increased prostate cancer risk: a pooled prospective study. *International Journal of Cancer.* 2004;108(3):418-424. https://doi.org/10.1002/ijc.11572

Sur, S., Panda, C. K. Molecular aspects of cancer chemopreventive and therapeutic efficacies of tea and tea polyphenols. *Nutrition.* 2017;43-44:8-15. https://doi.org/10.1016/j.nut.2017.06.006

Tappy, L. Le, K. Metabolic effects of fructose and the worldwide increase in obesity. *Physiological Review.* 2010;90:23-46. https://doi/10.1152/phyrev.00019.2009

Thivel, D., Tremblay, A., Genin, P. M., Panahi, S., Rivière, D., Duclos, M. Physical activity, inactivity, and sedentary behaviors: Definitions and implications in occupational health. *Frontiers in Public Health.* 2018;6:288. https://doi.org/10.3389/fpubh.2018.00288

Wagenlehner, F. M., Bschleipfer, T., Pilatz, A., Weidner, W. Pollen extract for chronic prostatitis-chronic pelvic pain syndrome. *Urology Clinic North America.* 2011;38(3):285-292. https://doi.org/10.1016/j.ucl.2011.04.004

Wei, J. T., Dunn, R., L., Sandler, H. M., McLaughlin, W., Montie, J. E., Litwin, M. S., et al. Comprehensive comparison of health-related quality of life after contemporary therapies for localized prostate cancer. *Journal of Clinical Oncology.* 2002; 20(2):557-566. https://doi.org/10.1200/JCO.2002.20.2.557

Wheless, J. History of the ketogenic diet. *Epilepsia.* 2008;49(Suppl. 8):3-5. https://doi.org/10.1111/j.1528-1167.2008.01821.x

Wheless, J. History and origin of the ketogenic diet. In C. E. Stafstrom and J. M. Rho (eds) *Epilepsy and the Ketogenic Diet.* 2008. (Totowa, NJ: Humana Press, Inc.) 31-50.

Wiederkehr, M., Krapf, R. Metabolic and endocrine effects of metabolic acidosis in humans. *Swiss Med Weekly.* 2001;131:127-132.

Wilt, T. J., MacDonald, R., Ishani, A. Beta-sitosterol for the treatment of benign prostatic hyperplasia: A Systemic review. *BJU International.* 1999;83(9):976-983.

Xu, G., Guan, L., Sun, J., Chen, Z.Y. Oxidation of cholesterol and Beta-sitosterol and prevention by natural antioxidants. *Journal of Agriculture and Food Chemistry.* 2009;57(19):9284-9292. https://doi.org/10.1021/jf902552s

Ying, M., Zhao, R., Jiang, D., Gu, S., Li, M. Lifestyle interventions to alleviate side effects on prostate cancer patients receiving androgen deprivation therapy: a meta-analysis. *Japanese Journal of Clinical Oncology.* 2018;48(9):827-834. https://doi.org/10.1093/jjco/hyy101

YuPeng, L., Fulan, H., DanDan, L., Fan, W., Lin, Z., WangYang, C., et al. Does physical activity reduce the risk of prostate cancer? A systematic review and meta-analysis. *European Urology.* 2011;60(5):1029-1044. https://doi.org/10.1016/j.eururo.2011.07.007

Norman RW, Coakes KE, Wright AS, Rittmaster RS. Androgen metabolism in men receiving finasteride before prostatectomy. J Urol. 1993;150:1736–1739 https://www.ncbi.nlm.nih.gov/pubmed/7692110

Gormley GJ, Stoner E, Bruskewitz RC, et al. The Effect of Finasteride in Men with Benign Prostatic Hyperplasia. The Finasteride Study Group. N Engl J Med. 1992; 327:1185–1191. http://www.nejm.org/doi/full/10.1056/NEJM199210223271701.

Thompson CA. Finasteride may Prevent Prostate Cancer. Am J Health Syst Pharm. 2003; 60:1511, 1515.

Persistent Sexual, Emotional, and Cognitive Impairment Post-Finasteride: A Survey of Men Reporting Symptoms, Christine Anne Ganzer, PhD, Alan Roy Jacobs, MD, and Farin Iqbal, https://doi.org/10.1177%2F1557988314538445

Kiguradze et al. (2017), Persistent erectile dysfunction in men exposed to the 5a-reductase inhibitors, finasteride, or dutasteride. PeerJ 5:e3020; DOI 10.7717/peerj.3020
https://peerj.com/articles/3020.pdf

McConnell JD, et col. The Effect of Finasteride on the Risk of Acute Urinary Retention and the Need for Surgical Treatment among Men with Benign Prostatic Hyperplasia. Finasteride Long-Term Efficacy and Safety Study Group. Engl J Med. 1998 Feb 26; 338(9):557-63. https://www.ncbi.nlm.nih.gov/pubmed/9475762.

Tammela TL et col. Urodynamic Effects of Finasteride in the Treatment of Bladder Outlet Obstruction due to Benign Prostatic Hyperplasia. J Urol. 1993 Feb; 149(2):342-4. https://www.ncbi.nlm.nih.gov/pubmed/7678871

Persistent Sexual, Emotional, and Cognitive Impairment Post-Finasteride: A Survey of Men Reporting Symptoms, Christine Anne Ganzer, PhD, Alan Roy Jacobs, MD, and Farin Iqbal,
https://doi.org/10.1177%2F1557988314538445

Kiguradze et al. (2017), Persistent erectile dysfunction in men exposed to the 5a-reductase inhibitors, finasteride, or dutasteride. PeerJ 5:e3020; DOI 10.7717/peerj.3020
https://peerj.com/articles/3020.pdf

Ramirez J. Severe hypotension Associated with α blocker Tamsulosin. BMJ. 2013 Nov 5;347: f6492.
https://www.ncbi.nlm.nih.gov/pubmed/24192968

Pärssinen O, Leppänen E, Keski-Rahkonen P, Mauriala T, Dugué B, Lehtonen M. Influence of Tamsulosin on the Iris and its Implications for Cataract Surgery. Investigative ophthalmology & visual science. 2006 Sep 1;47(9):3766-71.
https://www.ncbi.nlm.nih.gov/pubmed/16936084

Miah S, Catto J. BPH and Prostate Cancer Risk. Indian Journal of Urology: IJU: Journal of the Urological Society of India. 2014 Apr;30(2):214.
https://www.ncbi.nlm.nih.gov/pmc/articles/PMC3989826/

Roehrborn CG. Three Months' Treatment with the α 1-blocker Alfuzosin does not Affect Total or Transition Zone Volume of the Prostate. Prostate Cancer and Prostatic Diseases. 2006 Jun;9(2):121.
https://www.ncbi.nlm.nih.gov/pmc/articles/PMC1477612/

Wilt TJ, MacDonald R, Rutks I. Tamsulosin for Benign Prostatic Hyperplasia. Cochrane Database of Systematic Reviews (Online). 2003 (1). 1; 107(9):1426-31.
https://www.ncbi.nlm.nih.gov/pubmed/20927745

Montorsi F, Roehrborn C, Garcia-Penit J, Borre M, Roeleveld TA, Alimi JC, Gagnier P, Wilson TH. The Effects of Dutasteride or Tamsulosin alone and in Combination on Storage and Voiding Symptoms in Men with Lower Urinary Tract Symptoms (LUTS) and Benign Prostatic Hyperplasia (BPH): 4-year Data from the Combination of Avodart and Tamsulosin (CombAT) Study. BJU international. 2011 May
https://www.ncbi.nlm.nih.gov/pubmed/21348912

Roehrborn CG, Siami P, Barkin J, Damião R, Major-Walker K, Morrill B, Montorsi F. The Effects of Dutasteride, Tamsulosin and Combination Therapy on Lower Urinary Tract Symptoms in Men with Benign Prostatic Hyperplasia and Prostatic Enlargement: 2-year Results from the Combat Study. The Journal of Urology. 2008 Feb 1;179(2):616-21. https://www.ncbi.nlm.nih.gov/pubmed/18082216

Schulman CC, Lock TM, Buzelin JM, Boeminghaus F, Stephenson TP, Talja M. Long- term Use of Tamsulosin to Treat Lower Urinary Tract Symptoms/Benign Prostatic Hyperplasia. The Journal of Urology. 2001 Oct 1;166(4):1358-63.

https://www.ncbi.nlm.nih.gov/pubmed/11547074

Key, T J et al. "A case-control study of diet and prostate cancer" British journal of cancer vol. 76,5 (1997): 678-87.

Loic Le Marchand, Jean H. Hankin, Laurence N. Kolonel, Lynne R. Wilkens; Vegetable and Fruit Consumption in Relation to Prostate Cancer Risk in Hawaii: A Reevaluation of the Effect of Dietary Beta-Carotene, American Journal of Epidemiology, Volume 133, Issue 3, 1 February 1991, Pages 215–219, https://doi.org/10.1093/oxfordjournals.aje.a115865

Kazuko Yoshizawa, Walter C. Willett, Steven J. Morris, Meir J. Stampfer, Donna Spiegelman, Eric B. Rimm, Edward Giovannucci; Study of Prediagnostic Selenium Level in Toenails and the Risk of Advanced Prostate Cancer, JNCI: Journal of the National Cancer Institute, Volume 90, Issue 16, 19 August 1998, Pages 1219–1224, https://doi.org/10.1093/jnci/90.16.1219

Jennifer H. Cohen, Alan R. Kristal, Janet L. Stanford; Fruit and Vegetable Intakes and Prostate Cancer Risk, JNCI: Journal of the National Cancer Institute, Volume 92, Issue 1, 5 January 2000, Pages 61–68, https://doi.org/10.1093/jnci/92.1.61

Ann W. Hsing, George W. Comstock, Helen Abbey, B. Frank Polk; Serologic Precursors of Cancer. Retinol, Carotenoids, and Tocopherol and Risk of Prostate Cancer, JNCI: Journal of the National Cancer Institute, Volume 82, Issue 11, 6 June 1990, Pages 941–946, https://doi.org/10.1093/jnci/82.11.941

Neonatal Hormone Concentrations and Risk of Testicular Germ Cell Tumors (TGCT) Libby M. Morimoto, David Zava, Katherine A. McGlynn, Frank Z. Stanczyk, Alice Y. Kang, Xiaomei Ma, Joseph L. Wiemels and Catherine Metayer Cancer Epidemiol Biomarkers Prev April 1 2018 (27) (4) 488-495; DOI: 10.1158/1055-9965.EPI-17-0879

Dorai, T. , Cao, Y. , Dorai, B. , Buttyan, R. and Katz, A. E. (2001), Therapeutic potential of curcumin in human prostate cancer. III. Curcumin inhibits proliferation, induces apoptosis, and inhibits angiogenesis of LNCaP prostate cancer cells in vivo. Prostate, 47: 293-303. doi:10.1002/pros.1074

Phase II Randomized Clinical Trial of Lycopene Supplementation before Radical Prostatectomy Omer Kucuk, Fazlul H. Sarkar, Wael Sakr, Zora Djuric, Michael N. Pollak, Fred Khachik, Yi-Wei Li, Mousumi Banerjee, David Grignon, John S. Bertram, John D. Crissman, Edson J. Pontes and David P. Wood Jr. Cancer Epidemiol Biomarkers Prev August 1 2001 (10) (8) 861-868;

Di Silverio F, D'eramo G, Lubrano C, Flammia GP, Sciarra A, Palma E, Caponera M, Sciarra F. Evidence that Serenoa repens extract displays an antiestrogenic activity in prostatic tissue of benign prostatic hypertrophy patients. European urology. 1992;21:309-14.